Workouts For Dummies®

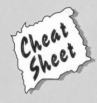

Cheat Sheet

W9-BNN-851

Keeping Yourself Motivated

- Make and keep commitments to yourself.
- Have faith in your body.
- Realize that you deserve to be fit and healthy.
- Enjoy increasing the strength of your body.
- Remember: You are getting healthier every day.

Starting Your First Workout Program

1. Motivate yourself to design and implement your own workout program.
2. Review the chapters on body types to figure out how your body responds to exercise (Chapters 5, 6, and 7).
3. Determine your fitness level with the tests provided in Chapter 8.
4. Scan the exercise chapters to find the exercises you want to put in your program. Add them to the chart in Appendix A.
5. Take your workouts on the road, to the office, or wherever you go.

Avoiding Injuries

Overtraining can lead to injuries. If you get injured, you're likely to quit exercising and never work out again. This isn't good. The following list helps you avoid unnecessary injuries. (See Chapter 4 for more information.)

- Watch for your body's warning signs and signals.
- Perform the exercises correctly. (Check the *Tips* and *Caution* sections after each exercise in this book.)
- Warm up and stretch before and after exercising.
- Start out slowly and gradually increase your workouts.
- Relax, breathe, and take time to enjoy your life.
- Get proper rest between exercise sessions.
- Use proper body mechanics when lifting objects or executing sports skills.
- Don't jump into an exercise too quickly.
- Don't overdo an activity.
- Don't exercise when you're ill or overtrained.
- Don't return to your normal exercise program until your athletic injuries have healed.

...For Dummies: Bestselling Book Series for Beginners

Workouts For Dummies®

Cheat
Sheet

Knowing Your Body Type

Researchers have found that human bodies have three distinct forms, called endomorphy, ectomorphy, and mesomorphy. Every person has one or more of the features of these body types, which make up how the body physically looks, reacts to exercise, and loses or gains weight. Each body type has specific characteristics, and anything in between the three main types is a blend of two types.

Figuring out which body type you have may be the first step in discovering your potential. Chapters 5, 6, and 7 give you a more thorough description of the typical characteristics of each of these types. After you have determined which body type most closely resembles your own, you can design a workout program to best suit your needs.

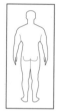

Meso

A mesomorph (or meso, for short) can be defined in one word . . . muscular. The well-developed, rectangular shapes of mesomorphs are representative of their thick bones and muscles. If you are a characteristic mesomorph, you have a well-defined chest and shoulders that are both larger and more broad than your waistline. Your abdomen is taut and your hips are narrow. Your buttocks, thighs, and calves are all toned and defined.

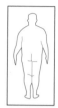

Ecto

A one-word description for the ectomorph body type (or ecto, for short) is slim. An ectomorph is relatively linear in shape with a delicate build, narrow hips and pelvis, and long arms and legs. As an ecto, your muscle and bone outlines are usually visible (especially if you are an extremely thin ecto), and you normally have less fat and muscle mass than people with other body types.

Endo

A one-word description of the endomorph body type (or endo, for short) is curvy. An endomorph body typically has the capacity for high fat storage. The majority of your body weight is either centered in the middle of your body or in your hip and buttocks regions. From top to bottom, your soft swelling curves create full, rounded shoulders, limbs, and a full trunk.

...For Dummies: Bestselling Book Series for Beginners

Praise For Workouts For Dummies

"I have never stuck with an exercise routine in my life until I started on Tamilee's program. She gave me a love for working out I never thought possible. Now it's grown into a more active lifestyle for me and my family. I look better and feel better. What a gift!!!
— Kimberly Hunter, newscaster ABC News San Diego

"I take my hat off to these accomplished fitness presenters, Tamilee and Lori, whose unique brand of lifestyle and fitness choices affect millions each day. Who would expect anything less from Tamilee — the creator of the original resistance exercise workout and the infamous Buns of Steel innovator? Her professional integrity and expertise will again prevail with this informative book and refreshing outlook — bringing her yet another well-deserved success. Congratulations!"
— Steve Block, President, SPRI Products, Inc.

"Whenever you try something new, you always need someone to introduce you to the terminology, slang words, and inside phrases that allow you to understand what you are doing and ask appropriate questions. No two people are better qualified than Tamilee Webb and Lori Seeger to answer your questions related to the entire physical fitness industry. This book proves invaluable in helping beginners and even seasoned exercise enthusiasts to gain the most from their exercise regimens."
— William W. Colvin, Ed.D, Professor of Kinesiology, California State University

"I have known Tamilee for 10 years — she lives for fitness and she lives for motivating others to be the best they can be! There are a lot of wannabe Tamilees, but you're getting the one and only! This book is simple, informative, and fun. You'll love it! DON'T QUIT!
— Jake Steinfeld, CEO of *Body By Jake,* and creator of Fit TV

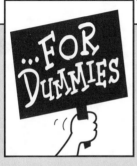
™

References for the Rest of Us!™

BESTSELLING BOOK SERIES FROM IDG

Do you find that traditional reference books are overloaded with technical details and advice you'll never use? Do you postpone important life decisions because you just don't want to deal with them? Then our *...For Dummies*® business and general reference book series is for you.

...For Dummies business and general reference books are written for those frustrated and hard-working souls who know they aren't dumb, but find that the myriad of personal and business issues and the accompanying horror stories make them feel helpless. *...For Dummies* books use a lighthearted approach, a down-to-earth style, and even cartoons and humorous icons to diffuse fears and build confidence. Lighthearted but not lightweight, these books are perfect survival guides to solve your everyday personal and business problems.

> *"More than a publishing phenomenon, 'Dummies' is a sign of the times."*
>
> — The New York Times

> *"A world of detailed and authoritative information is packed into them..."*
>
> — U.S. News and World Report

> *"...you won't go wrong buying them."*
>
> — Walter Mossberg, Wall Street Journal, on IDG Books' ...For Dummies books

Already, millions of satisfied readers agree. They have made *...For Dummies* the #1 introductory level computer book series and a best-selling business book series. They have written asking for more. So, if you're looking for the best and easiest way to learn about business and other general reference topics, look to *...For Dummies* to give you a helping hand.

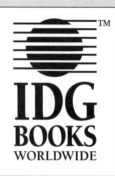

IDG
BOOKS
WORLDWIDE

WORKOUTS
FOR
DUMMIES®

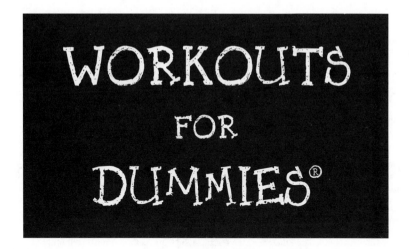

by Tamilee Webb
with Lori Seeger

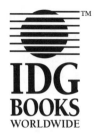

IDG Books Worldwide, Inc.
An International Data Group Company

Foster City, CA ♦ Chicago, IL ♦ Indianapolis, IN ♦ New York, NY

Workouts For Dummies®

Published by
IDG Books Worldwide, Inc.
An International Data Group Company
919 E. Hillsdale Blvd.
Suite 400
Foster City, CA 94404
www.idgbooks.com (IDG Books Worldwide Web site)
www.dummies.com (Dummies Press Web site)

Library of Congress Catalog Card No.: 98-88737

ISBN: 0-7645-5124-8

Printed in the United States of America

10 9 8 7 6 5 4 3 2 1

1O/QS/RS/ZY/IN

Distributed in the United States by IDG Books Worldwide, Inc.

Distributed by Macmillan Canada for Canada; by Transworld Publishers Limited in the United Kingdom; by IDG Norge Books for Norway; by IDG Sweden Books for Sweden; by Woodslane Pty. Ltd. for Australia; by Woodslane (NZ) Ltd. for New Zealand; by Addison Wesley Longman Singapore Pte Ltd. for Singapore, Malaysia, Thailand, and Indonesia; by Norma Comunicaciones S.A. for Colombia; by Intersoft for South Africa; by International Thomson Publishing for Germany, Austria and Switzerland; by Distribuidora Cuspide for Argentina; by Livraria Cultura for Brazil; by Ediciencia S.A. for Ecuador; by Ediciones ZETA S.C.R. Ltda. for Peru; by WS Computer Publishing Corporation, Inc., for the Philippines; by Contemporanea de Ediciones for Venezuela; by Express Computer Distributors for the Caribbean and West Indies; by Micronesia Media Distributor, Inc. for Micronesia; by Grupo Editorial Norma S.A. for Guatemala; by Chips Computadoras S.A. de C.V. for Mexico; by Editorial Norma de Panama S.A. for Panama; by Wouters Import for Belgium; by American Bookshops for Finland. Authorized Sales Agent: Anthony Rudkin Associates for the Middle East and North Africa.

For general information on IDG Books Worldwide's books in the U.S., please call our Consumer Customer Service department at 800-762-2974. For reseller information, including discounts and premium sales, please call our Reseller Customer Service department at 800-434-3422.

For information on where to purchase IDG Books Worldwide's books outside the U.S., please contact our International Sales department at 317-596-5530 or fax 317-596-5692.

For information on foreign language translations, please contact our Foreign & Subsidiary Rights department at 650-655-3021 or fax 650-655-3281.

For sales inquiries and special prices for bulk quantities, please contact our Sales department at 650-655-3200 or write to the address above.

For information on using IDG Books Worldwide's books in the classroom or for ordering examination copies, please contact our Educational Sales department at 800-434-2086 or fax 317-596-5499.

For press review copies, author interviews, or other publicity information, please contact our Public Relations department at 650-655-3000 or fax 650-655-3299.

For authorization to photocopy items for corporate, personal, or educational use, please contact Copyright Clearance Center, 222 Rosewood Drive, Danvers, MA 01923, or fax 978-750-4470.

is a trademark under exclusive license to IDG Books Worldwide, Inc., from International Data Group, Inc.

About the Authors

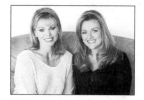 **Tamilee Webb** (MA) is best known for her video success series "Buns of Steel." Her bachelor of arts degree in physical education and master of arts degree in exercise science, from California State University, Chico, place Tamilee on the cutting edge of fitness education. She is continually developing, promoting, and producing the most innovative programs for fitness fans everywhere.

After 22 award winning Buns of Steel titles, Tamilee has developed her personal line: Tamilee's Building Tighter Assets, Abs Abs Abs, and Toning Mind and Body. You can find these and more on her Web page www.tamileewebb.com.

Along with video productions, Tamilee has co-hosted *ESPN Fitness Pros* and is currently co-hosting Fox Sports *FiT TV* with Jake Steinfeld on television. If you have ever channel surfed, you have seen Tamilee host Guthy-Renker Fitness "Perfect Abs" and "Turbo Glider" equipment.

Tamilee's first book, *The Original Rubber Band Workout,* was released in 1986 and is now sold in six countries and five languages. This was followed by her second book, *Step Up Fitness,* which was released in 1994.

Named 1993's "Fitness Instructor of the Year" by IDEA, the Association of Fitness Professionals, Tamilee's other honors include *Self Magazine's* 1992 award for "Best Lower Body Exercise Video" for Buns of Steel 3; second runner-up for "Ms. Fitness America" in 1991; California State University Chico "Outstanding Alumni" in 1990 and 1996; and IDEA's "Best Exercise Video" in 1987.

Lori Seeger (MA) moved to California after receiving her bachelor of science degree in business and marketing from the State University of New York at Buffalo. Since then she has received a professional certificate in exercise science and fitness instruction from the University of California, San Diego and is completing her master of arts degree in psychology from the University for Humanistic Studies.

She is the writer of this book and has been working with Tamilee Webb as her right-hand person for over seven years assisting in the development of Webb International associated fitness programs and products. In addition to her experience in television and video production, she has also appeared with Tamilee on *FiT TV* as well as several fitness videos and infomercials. Lori is also a fitness instructor and personal trainer in San Diego, CA.

ABOUT IDG BOOKS WORLDWIDE

Welcome to the world of IDG Books Worldwide.

IDG Books Worldwide, Inc., is a subsidiary of International Data Group, the world's largest publisher of computer-related information and the leading global provider of information services on information technology. IDG was founded more than 30 years ago by Patrick J. McGovern and now employs more than 9,000 people worldwide. IDG publishes more than 290 computer publications in over 75 countries. More than 90 million people read one or more IDG publications each month.

Launched in 1990, IDG Books Worldwide is today the #1 publisher of best-selling computer books in the United States. We are proud to have received eight awards from the Computer Press Association in recognition of editorial excellence and three from Computer Currents' First Annual Readers' Choice Awards. Our best-selling *...For Dummies*® series has more than 50 million copies in print with translations in 31 languages. IDG Books Worldwide, through a joint venture with IDG's Hi-Tech Beijing, became the first U.S. publisher to publish a computer book in the People's Republic of China. In record time, IDG Books Worldwide has become the first choice for millions of readers around the world who want to learn how to better manage their businesses.

Our mission is simple: Every one of our books is designed to bring extra value and skill-building instructions to the reader. Our books are written by experts who understand and care about our readers. The knowledge base of our editorial staff comes from years of experience in publishing, education, and journalism — experience we use to produce books to carry us into the new millennium. In short, we care about books, so we attract the best people. We devote special attention to details such as audience, interior design, use of icons, and illustrations. And because we use an efficient process of authoring, editing, and desktop publishing our books electronically, we can spend more time ensuring superior content and less time on the technicalities of making books.

You can count on our commitment to deliver high-quality books at competitive prices on topics you want to read about. At IDG Books Worldwide, we continue in the IDG tradition of delivering quality for more than 30 years. You'll find no better book on a subject than one from IDG Books Worldwide.

IDG
BOOKS
WORLDWIDE

John Kilcullen
Chairman and CEO
IDG Books Worldwide, Inc.

Steven Berkowitz
President and Publisher
IDG Books Worldwide, Inc.

*Eighth Annual
Computer Press
Awards ≥ 1992*

*Ninth Annual
Computer Press
Awards ≥ 1993*

*Tenth Annual
Computer Press
Awards ≥ 1994*

*Eleventh Annual
Computer Press
Awards ≥ 1995*

Dedication

From Tamilee:

This book is dedicated to the love of my life, my husband Paul E. Chasan. He has offered me so much of his knowledge and support to help me develop this book. Thank you for your understanding, your love, and walking our dogs Kassie and Sparky while I was so busy with the book.

Author's Acknowledgments

From Tamilee:

It takes many talented people to dedicate their time and effort, not to mention endless amounts of energy, to put together a book. I know, you thought I did this all myself, right? I would like to introduce to you my friends, family, and associates who have helped make *Workouts For Dummies* possible. Thank you all from the bottom of my Buns of Steel.

Lori Seeger, who in the past seven years has gone from employee to business partner to friend to little sister. There is nothing you couldn't accomplish that your heart wanted, and now as a writer, you are one step closer to your dreams. I thank you personally "Lur" for your support, travel stories, sisterly love, and dedication to writing *Workouts For Dummies* while planning your wedding and going to school. You did it and did it well.

A special thank-you to Tom Fahey, Ph.D., one of my great professors at California State University, Chico. I appreciate your time and expertise as the technical advisor for *Workouts For Dummies*. Your superb teaching skills and the information you have shared in the books you've written have been admired by your students and peers for many years. Now consumers can benefit from your knowledge as well. This was an assignment I enjoyed handing in to you for your feedback — probably because I didn't have to be graded on it. Thank you!

I wish to thank my physician and friend, Dianna Rosenberg, M.D., for her assistance, knowledge, and suggestions for the pregnancy workout and guidelines. You're the only doctor that gives me a great ab workout during my appointment . . . you keep me laughing.

When humor is nowhere to be found while writing the technical information, who do you call upon? Your girlfriends of course. Together, we seem to find a way of making anything funny. Mindy Marinos, Kelley Stimpel Rasmussen, and Debbie MacLean Rider came to the rescue by adding their special touches. Thank you all for making my abs ache from the joy of laughter.

Thank goodness for make-up artists like Yvonne Ouellette. Without her expertise, I would probably look more like Tammy Faye than Tamilee at the end of my workout. Thank you for making me look and feel beautiful on all my shoots.

Many thanks to Shari Turner for her share in helping type up all those exercises. She knows them all too well from our many shows on FiT TV.

And finally, thank you to everyone at IDG Books especially Bill Helling, project editor and Stacey Mickelbart, copy editor, for their input, suggestions, and sense of humor in editing this book. Many thanks to Stacy Collins for rejecting my first book proposal and seeing my future in authoring *Workouts For Dummies.* Thank you for the wonderful opportunity.

From Lori:

I first want to thank Tamilee for giving me the opportunity to work with her on this project. Being both my friend and boss, we have shared many years of laughter and success through teamwork. She has offered me guidance on topics from career endeavors to boyfriends and continually given me her love in every aspect of my life. People have stopped us many times to ask us if we are sisters. We may not be biological sisters but we are surely soul sisters.

I'm grateful to the entire IDG Books staff for their assistance and hard work with special thanks to Stacy Collins, Bill Helling, and Stacey Mickelbart.

To my family and friends, I owe a great deal of appreciation for their unceasing love and support. I would like to give special thanks to my Aunt Sharon, my father Tom, and my grandmother Millie (who will always remain in my heart) for their endless love and encouragement. To my mother Judith, I dedicate my first writing experience, for she is the one who continuously inspires me, believes in me, and has been there for me. Most of all I want to thank her for showing me the beauty of the sunsets, the moon, the clouds, and the storms.

Finally, I want to thank my fiancé Richard Biggers for his support, wisdom, and compassion. He has taught me the true meaning of passion and unconditional love, and it is with him that I have discovered what life is really about.

Publisher's Acknowledgments

We're proud of this book; please register your comments through our IDG Books Worldwide Online Registration Form located at http://my2cents.dummies.com.

Some of the people who helped bring this book to market include the following:

Acquisitions, Editorial, and Media Development

Project Editor: Bill Helling

Acquisitions Editor: Stacy S. Collins

Copy Editor: Stacey Mickelbart

Technical Editor: Dr. Tom Fahey, Ph.D.

Media Development Editor: Marita Ellixson

Associate Permissions Editor: Carmen Krikorian

Editorial Manager: Kelly Ewing

Editorial Assistant: Paul E. Kuzmic

Production

Project Coordinator: Valery Bourke

Layout and Graphics: Lou Boudreau, Linda M. Boyer, Angela F. Hunckler, Brent Savage, Jacque Schneider, Kate Snell, Brian Torwelle

Proofreaders: Christine Berman, Michelle Croninger, Sharon Duffy, Nancy Price, Rebecca Senninger, Janet M. Withers

Indexer: Sherry Massey

General and Administrative

IDG Books Worldwide, Inc.: John Kilcullen, CEO; Steven Berkowitz, President and Publisher

IDG Books Technology Publishing: Brenda McLaughlin, Senior Vice President and Group Publisher

Dummies Technology Press and Dummies Editorial: Diane Graves Steele, Vice President and Associate Publisher; Mary Bednarek, Director of Acquisitions and Product Development; Kristin A. Cocks, Editorial Director

Dummies Trade Press: Kathleen A. Welton, Vice President and Publisher; Kevin Thornton, Acquisitions Manager

IDG Books Production for Dummies Press: Michael R. Britton, Vice President of Production and Creative Services; Cindy L. Phipps, Manager of Project Coordination, Production Proofreading, and Indexing; Kathie S. Schutte, Supervisor of Page Layout; Shelley Lea, Supervisor of Graphics and Design; Debbie J. Gates, Production Systems Specialist; Robert Springer, Supervisor of Proofreading; Debbie Stailey, Special Projects Coordinator; Tony Augsburger, Supervisor of Reprints and Bluelines

Dummies Packaging and Book Design: Robin Seaman, Creative Director; Kavish + Kavish, Cover Design

♦

The publisher would like to give special thanks to Patrick J. McGovern, without whom this book would not have been possible.

Contents at a Glance

Cartoons at a Glance

By Rich Tennant

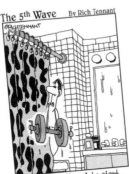

page 5

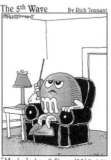

page 57

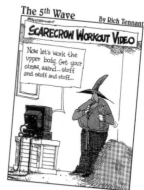

page 107

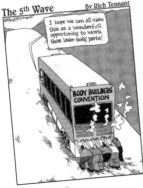

page 159

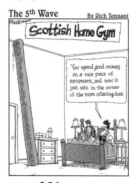

page 201

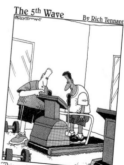

page 299

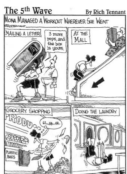

page 317

Fax: 978-546-7747 • E-mail: the5wave@tiac.net

Table of Contents

Introduction

• •

*E*very few months a new diet, wonder drug, or workout machine hits the market and consumers spend billions of dollars searching for the quick fix that results in a physically fit body. Promises of shedding pounds and instantaneously toning tummies and thighs mislead many of us to believe that good health can be ordered from television shows and catalogs. Unfortunately, no product or pill can give you a healthy, fit body — you must be willing to dedicate *yourself* to that goal.

The secret to good health is actually very basic: Eat a healthy diet, exercise, rest your body, and do your best to find balance in all aspects of your life.

Now that you realize you may actually have to work to get what you want, you're ready to get started. You may be the type of person who is easily motivated and jumps into a workout head first — not coming up for air unless you're injured. Or, you may hate exercising and think that beads of sweat on your brow are repulsive. Whether you're at one of these extremes or somewhere in between, you can find tons of information in this book to help you create a challenging, yet comfortable, workout program. You can figure out how to determine your body type and your level of physical conditioning, as well as various ways to work out at home, on the road, at the office, or on a boring date.

If you give yourself a chance by making exercise a part of your lifestyle, your body will reward you. Remember, no such thing as a perfect body exists, but you can endeavor to have perfect balance between your mind, body, and self.

How to Use This Book

You can skip around from chapter to chapter learning new exercises or pieces of eye-opening information, but you'll get the best results by:

1. Getting yourself motivated to design and implement your own workout program. (Part I)

2. Reviewing the chapters on the different body types and figuring out how your body best responds to exercise. (Part II)

3. Determining your fitness level with the simple tests provided in Chapter 8. (Part II)

4. Scanning the exercise chapters and finding the exercises you want to put in your program. (Parts III and IV)

5. Taking your workouts on the road or to the office. (Part V)

Whether you're a beginner or an advanced exerciser, you can find valuable information and innovative exercise techniques that help keep exercise a fun part of your lifestyle.

How This Book Is Organized

Workouts For Dummies is organized into seven parts, and the chapters within give you detailed information or exercises on the part topics. You may notice that I refer you to various chapters as you are reading if more in-depth information is provided elsewhere in the book on that topic. The following overview of the seven parts shows you what you can find where.

Part I: Getting Started

Don't skip over Chapter 1, which is about motivation. I firmly believe that in order to implement exercise into your lifestyle you *have to want to do it*. If I can get you mentally psyched up to work out, you'll be better able to get your body moving. After you're motivated, I tell you what clothes and shoes are best for the various workouts, how to listen to your body's aches and pains so that you can avoid injuries, and how to warm up, cool down, and stretch when you're starting and finishing off your workouts.

Part II: My Body Type's Best Workout

Part II gives you an opportunity to figure out what type of body you have. Cut out a picture of yourself and match it up to the mesomorph, ectomorph, or endomorph body shapes on the scale. I also give you tests to determine your fitness level and create a workout program specifically designed for your body.

Part III: Upper-Body Workouts

Get your heart and upper-body muscles moving in Part III. I give you tips on choosing cardiovascular exercises and the best exercises for burning calories. You can start pumping up your arms, chest, back, and abdominals with a variety of upper-body muscle-conditioning exercises. Pick and choose your favorite exercises to put in your personal workout program.

Part IV: Lower-Body Workouts

Buns, legs, and thighs are covered in Part IV. If you're looking to tone and tighten your lower body, you won't find a how-to guide on liposuction here, but you can find several exercises to shape up your muscles. I give you my personal favorite bun strengtheners, like squats and lunges, as well as a few stories about how I got into shape.

Part V: Special Workouts at Home, on the Road, in the Office, or at the Gym

Part V gives you workout options whether you're at work, at home, or on the road. I also included some options for cardiovascular workouts when you're traveling, plus tips on selecting a gym that meets your workout needs. You're left with no excuse to avoid working out after reading these chapters. You even find specialty workouts with bands and tubes, plus programs for seniors and moms-to-be.

Part VI: The Part of Tens

The Part of Tens is your resource for great information on health and fitness. I list my ten favorite videos, which I happen to be the creator of, plus my ten favorite fitness books, and my favorite exercises.

Part VII: Appendixes

This part has an appendix containing an exercise program chart that you can personalize to fit your own needs. You can also find an appendix listing great workout sites on the Web.

Icons Used in This Book

Tip: Tips give you additional advice on a topic or specific information on how to best perform an exercise.

Myth Buster: The Myth Buster man reveals all the false information people have conjured up over the years about exercise and what it can or can't do for you.

Advanced Stuff: If you want to throw out a few exercise science terms at your next cocktail party, read up on the advanced stuff. This icon provides you with in-depth knowledge on the topic being discussed.

Author's Pick: Throughout the book I mention a few of my favorite books and products you may find interesting and helpful. They have all been *Tamilee tested* for endurance and reliability.

Caution: The caution icon gives you specific information on performing each exercise and what to watch for to help you avoid injuries.

Lingo: This icon points out workout terms that you should know because you'll see them time and time again.

Tamilee Says: Just another icon (with bits and pieces of priceless information, of course) that we threw in so that I could have the illustrators make a caricature of my head. Pretty cool, huh?

Getting Started

For most of us, getting started is the hardest part. If you're already in the habit of *not* exercising, you may find that you have to train yourself into a new habit of good health. In fact, if you break it down, fitness is simply a good habit. As we grow up we learn to do certain things to take care of ourselves like brushing our teeth or eating three meals a day. Your internal health is just as vital — and by creating a habit of exercising your body, you not only prolong your longevity, you also enhance your years by avoiding illness, increase your energy and ability to be more active, and find new ways to enjoy life. It's never too late to pick up a new habit — so get started now.

Part I
Getting Started

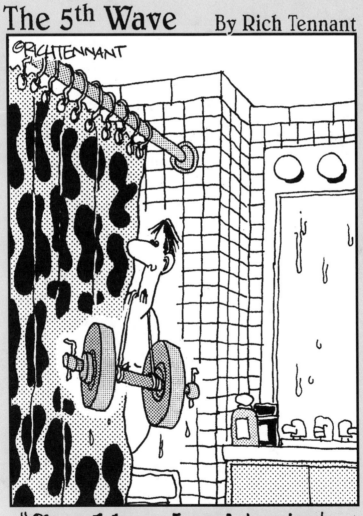

The 5th Wave   By Rich Tennant

"Okay, I know I need to start working out. Now, can I please have my soap-on-a-rope back?"

In this part . . .

My first goal is to get you motivated to work out, and motivation is what you can find in this leading part. After you have the desire and drive to get your buns in shape, I help you get suited up for working out. I give you a mini-education on fitness shoes so you can determine what type of foot you have and which shoes best meet your needs. You also get tips on how to find the best place in your home to do your workouts and what to wear while you're exercising in different climates. Don't think that I expect you to get injured, but I give you some prevention tips to help you avoid typical fitness-related injuries. By this point you're ready to begin, so I give you information on how best to warm up, cool down, and stretch your body before and after your workouts.

Chapter 1

Motivate Your Mind, Exercise Your Body

. . . .

In This Chapter

▶ Motivating your mind

▶ Balancing your mind, body, and self

▶ Discovering the origin of your genes

▶ Checking out body types

. . . .

1 love to motivate people. It gives me great pleasure to know that many people are trying to develop healthier lifestyles. Through the years, the most popular question at my lectures is, "Why can't I look like . . . ." This question is a thought many of us have at one time or another. I wish I could tell you that you can look like anyone you want to, but the fact is, you have a body unique to you, and you can only work to make your body the best it can be. Too often, people who decide to work out pick someone else's body image and work out as hard as they can to attain it, but when they don't attain this goal, they get frustrated and give up. Before setting your sights on having Demi Moore's physique or Sylvester Stallone's body, take a look at the genetic characteristics your parents gave you. Determining your body type is important to developing a workout program that best suits your needs.

What Your Health Means to You

Your health is the most valuable thing you possess. Most of us take our health for granted and think that bad things won't happen to us. When you're a teenager, you rarely worry about heart disease, diabetes, or arthritis. In fact, many of us abuse our bodies, assuming they'll just snap back into shape the way they did when we were kids. If you've already entered your adult years, you probably know that this isn't the case. If aging gracefully is your goal, you need to take care of both your internal and external health.

Leading a healthy lifestyle takes about the same amount of commitment as brushing your teeth, showering, and getting dressed in the morning. If you can find time in your daily schedule to groom yourself, why not take the same amount of time to become healthier? If you make that commitment to yourself and live it each day, you can get healthy.

Avoiding the wrong attitude

If you're the average person, you may assume that you're a healthy individual because you've never had any serious injuries or illnesses, don't drink or smoke, and only occasionally indulge in junk food. Your weekly exercise may consist of taking out the trash and watching ESPN's SportsCenter. One morning you wake up and find that your legs won't move, you can't get out of bed or walk to the kitchen, and taking out the trash is definitely out of the picture. After consulting with your doctor, you're told that your muscles don't work anymore because you didn't take care of them or use their full potential. The doctor asks you when you last went for a walk, played a game of baseball, or stretched your muscles. Unfortunately, you can't remember. You just assumed your health would always be fine and that exercise was only for "those people" who want to show off their bodies or need to lose weight.

Fortunately, this is a make-believe story, but it represents the attitudes many of us have regarding our health. Many times something bad has to happen before we wake up and realize that we're taking advantage of our bodies and our health. Using your mind and learning how to care for your body are the first and most important steps in maintaining a healthy life.

Motivating your mind

Have you ever talked yourself into doing something? Maybe you've tried psyching yourself up to ask the girl next door for a date, get your buns out of bed at 5 a.m. to work out, or finish a project that you're procrastinating on. After you've set your mind, your body follows through. But before you decide to do anything, you must have desire. Desire is what motivates your mind.

Think of advertising, for example. How many times have you watched a commercial for food and then began feeling hungry? Advertising is a way of creating a desire to buy. Whether the ad is for food, cars, or exercise equipment, if the product or the idea appeals to your mind, you'll desire that product. The infomercial industry in particular has capitalized on our desires. If you watch any exercise equipment infomercial, you'll find they're full of hype, testimonials, and lots of promises.

Making muscles and losing fat

If making muscle isn't a good enough reason to get your butt in gear and start your new workout program, I can give you a little more incentive. Muscle helps your body *burn fat!* Hello, did you hear me? Yes, I said burn fat. Most of us like to burn off a little now and then, especially after dining on a fine piece of "Death By Chocolate" dessert. Now you're probably wondering, "What in the world do my muscles do to help my body burn fat?" The answer is easy. Your muscles are live tissue and need fuel to grow. They receive a portion of their fuel from the fat stored in your body. As you continue to exercise aerobically and do resistance training, your muscles grow, and they'll need more fuel, also known as fat.

Infomercials motivate you to get in shape, so you buy the featured product. Right after you watch the show, you're pumped up and ready to work out. Unfortunately, six weeks later when your product arrives, you've forgotten why you liked it, and you probably aren't feeling very motivated to use it. You wanted the product and now you have it, so what's missing? It's the desire to use it. Getting in shape is possible only if you stay committed to your goals of exercising, eating right, and taking care of your mind and body.

As a fitness specialist, my goal is to feed your mind with information that inspires you to exercise your body. But even if I tell you all the benefits of exercise, the bottom line is that *you* have to want to do it. You've already taken the first step by picking up this book. You may be looking for a plan of action, or perhaps you're already in action and need a little pepping up. In either case, as long as you continue to fuel your mind with the desire to have a healthy body, you can keep your body moving. Just stick with me.

Remaining consistent

Did you know that if you do something consistently for over 30 days it becomes a habit? It's true. For example, after a month of putting on your seat belt when you get in a car, clicking your belt becomes habitual. So why not make exercise a habit? Try it out. Set a goal to take 15 minutes out of each day to exercise. Be consistent and stick to your promise for 30 to 45 days. I'm not a gambler, but I bet you'll begin to develop a healthy habit of exercising.

Too Much Can Put You Out of Balance

Sometimes people take a good thing and overdo it. I remember thinking as a kid, "Well if it's good for me, more of it must be better." This philosophy is not always true. In fact, too much of a good thing can create something bad. For instance, vitamin A is good for you, but a daily overdose can cause dermatitis. Too much exercise isn't going to give you skin problems, but too much exercise *may* cause injury. This is where the idea of *balance* comes in. Having a balanced lifestyle is something most of us need to work on. Look at the pyramid of life in Figure 1-1.

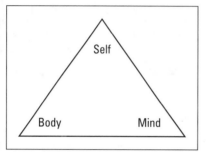

Figure 1-1:
The pyramid of life illustrates a balanced lifestyle.

Our lives are meant to be balanced, but most of us tilt to one side or the other by putting too much time and energy into one particular aspect.

The mind

The mind is a complex and powerful part of the balanced pyramid, constantly craving stimulation and knowledge. Keeping this part of your pyramid in balance can be accomplished in a variety of ways, such as reading books and newspapers, watching educational television, going to school, or traveling. Whatever your goals are, you should try to keep your mental focus. Starting a fitness program, for example, can be frustrating because you don't always see the results of your hard work right away. By having faith in yourself and keeping your mind motivated toward your goal, you'll reap the rewards. A healthy mind brings forth favorable action, which can positively affect your body and self.

The body

Having a balanced body means you're healthy both internally and externally. It's easy to sometimes neglect what you can't see — like your lungs, heart, liver, and stomach. If you could look in the mirror and see what your body looked like on the inside, you would probably stop indulging bad habits like smoking and eating a donut a day, and start exercising instead. But for now you can only view your external health, which at times may be deceiving.

Judging someone's body from what you see on the outside can be just as misleading as judging a book by its cover. You have no idea if what's inside is good or not. Just because someone appears slim doesn't mean he or she is healthy. Creating a balanced body means taking care of your internal health first. By taking care of your organs, muscles, and bones you'll be rewarded with a fit and vibrant exterior.

The self

Your inner self is very personal and for many people, private. I perceive this valuable part of our being as a key to true balance in life. The self envelops three categories of your life: your work, your family, and your personal development.

Most of us spend more time at work than with our families or on self-improvement. Fast forward your life until a few moments before your death and ask yourself, "What do I wish I'd spent more time in my life doing?" Do you think your answer would be "working"? I doubt it. So why take the chance of regretting how you spend the days and years of your life? Think of your inner self as a separate pyramid; in each corner you must devote equal time and energy to your life's work, your family and friends, and your personal self-development (as shown in Figure 1-2). After you find balance within yourself, you'll be better able to find balance in your life pyramid, too.

Figure 1-2:
Try to balance all three aspects of the self pyramid.

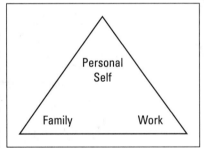

Who Gave Me These Genes?

Have you ever wished you looked more like someone else? Maybe you crave a body similar to John Kennedy Jr.'s, or Cindy Crawford's. Or maybe you just wish you had long legs or a rippled stomach. I have asked people this question a lot, and just about every one of them has told me that they have one or more body parts they wish they could change. I'm right in line with all of you. At times I have thought to myself, "If only I could have her legs, or her butt, I would . . ." I finally stopped and asked myself, "I would what?" Be happier? It took some time, but I now realize that I should be grateful for what I have: a fit and healthy body. All I need to do is keep it healthy. I've changed my "If only I had" statement to "Thou shalt work with thy body, not against it."

So who gave you that body anyway? No, it wasn't the person who invented ice cream — it was your parents. They didn't have a choice in the genes they passed on to you. Upon conception, your parents' DNA designates the characteristics chosen for your body makeup. It's kind of like a slot machine — you just get what you get. Your job is to take what you have been given and keep it healthy and fit.

From the color of your eyes to the length of your neck, your genes predetermine all of your features. This includes how short or tall you are, the type of musculature you are able to develop, and which parts of your body are most likely to carry fat. Take a look at the bodies of your parents and grandparents. That may give you a little insight on how your own body develops. You can thank mom and dad for better or worse. Maybe you got lucky with that cute little button nose, but then maybe you got a nose like Cyrano de Bergerac.

DNA and you

DNA (deoxyribonucleic acid) is the blueprint for the makeup of your body. Each chain of DNA that codes for a characteristic of your body is called a gene. A gene directs the body's cellular machinery to produce certain proteins. These proteins can be structural, such as collagen, or direct the manufacture of other body components like enzymes. They also regulate processes such as your appetite, energy use, and muscle mass.

At the time of conception, your DNA gets put into a random lottery in which certain genes or traits are expressed. This process doesn't know what the current fashion trends are so a body that may have been a blessing a 100 years ago may be a curse today. The fact is your parents' genes go into a biological blender and what comes out is a mixture of their best and, yes, worst, traits. The good news is that many of the characteristics that were designed by your genes, such as tendency to gain weight in your mid-section or being prone to heart disease, can be overcome if you make the choice to lead a healthy lifestyle by exercising and eating right.

So if you are thinking of blaming your parents entirely for what you look like because you don't like what you've got, think again. It's your responsibility to take what you were given and make the most of it. I was given a round butt and it's up to me to keep it toned, fit, and strong. Long, lean legs will only be in my dreams, but that doesn't mean I can't keep them toned and throw on a pair of high heels when I'm trying to look taller. My motto is, "Exercise and improvise."

TAMILEE SAYS

Keeping yourself motivated

When I'm feeling a little down and need motivation to get my spirits back up, I turn to positive affirmations. Affirmations are short, simple statements that get right to the point and go straight to the heart. Surely you've had some days where just a few kind words can take you from one end of the spectrum to the other. The following are some of my favorite affirmations related to health and the body. (I like to keep a copy of my favorites in my wallet so I can read them when I need a little lift in my spirits.)

Make and keep commitments to yourself.

I have faith in my body.

I deserve to be fit and healthy.

I am happy, healthy, and fit.

My body is in harmony with the universe.

I enjoy increasing my body's strength.

I am getting healthier every day.

My body is important to my everyday work.

My body mirrors my inner thoughts.

My body radiates health and energy.

My mind is clear; my body is fit.

To achieve, you must believe.

Take action today and live it forever.

Take care of your body and it will take care of you.

If you don't use it, you lose it.

Health is a gift some people don't notice until it's too late.

What's Your Make and Model?

LINGO

All cars are categorized into body types like economy, compact, mid-size, and luxury, so why not categorize human bodies by types? You can — and the scientific word for body types is *somatotypes*. Researchers have found that human somatotypes have three distinct characteristics, called endomorphy, ectomorphy, and mesomorphy (see Chapters 5, 6, and 7 for more in-depth descriptions). Every person has one or more of the characteristics of these body types, which make up how the body physically looks, reacts to exercise, and loses or gains weight. As you can see on the scale in Figure 1-3, each body type has specific characteristics, and anything in between the three main types is a blend of two types.

Now that you're motivated and committed to exercising, eating right, spending quality time with your family, and reserving a little quiet time for yourself, you're ready to take action and start shaping up your body. Staying dedicated to these goals gives you the ability to reach your potential.

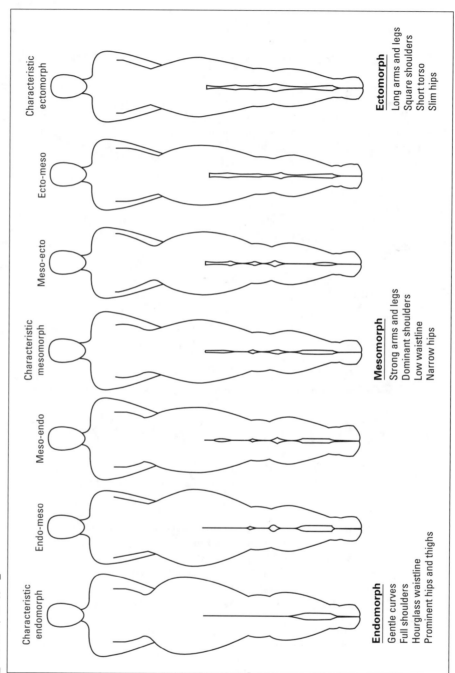

Figure 1-3:
Can you
find your
make and
model?

Your first step is figuring out what you have to start with. This is your reality check. Figuring out which body type you have (see Chapters 5, 6, and 7) may be the first step in discovering your potential. First, review the scale in Figure 1-3, and select a body shape that most resembles your own. Label this shape **R**. Next, select a body shape that you would ideally like to have and label it **I**. Are your two shapes on opposite ends of the scale or are they within one or two body types of each other? If your ideal (I) body type on the opposite end of the scale from your realistic(R) body type? Now look at the types between your I and R marks. Choosing to achieve a body type within one or two types of your realistic is a good, reasonable range within which to set your goal.

Pick the body type that is in this reasonable range (between your I and R) and label it **P**. This indicates your potential. The ability to make great changes in your body is possible if you stay committed to your goal. Rather than being satisfied with reality, try to realize your potential and go for it!

Body type geometry

In the past, names like pear, apple, stick, or carrot were used to describe body shapes. I don't know many guys who want to be referred to as a pear, and I think the days of women wanting a stick-like figure went out with Twiggy. I have read and heard other fitness professionals describe human body shapes using geometric shapes like cones, rulers, and pyramids. They seem to make more sense than the fruit metaphors, and they aren't as humiliating. Each one of the shapes represents where the body carries most of its weight. This weight may consist of primarily fat or muscle, or a good balance of both. For example, the cone shape represents a body that tends to gain weight from the waist up. The opposite of the cone is the pyramid figure.

This body carries most of its weight from the hips on down. The hourglass figure has a broad chest and shoulders, a narrow waist, and hips that are symmetrical with the shoulders. Take a look at the various body types in Figure 1-3. The list in this sidebar matches the geometric shapes with these body parts.

Which shape most describes your body type? Use your knowledge of somatotypes to better serve your body's needs when working out. Not all workouts or exercises are appropriate for every body type, but all of us share the need to move our muscles. Regardless of your body shape, to stay in shape you need to train your body with cardiovascular, strengthening, and flexibility exercises.

Shape	Body type
Ruler	Ectomorph
Cone	Ecto-meso
Hourglass	Mesomorph
Pyramid	Meso-endo
Spoon	Endomorph

Chapters 5, 6, and 7 give you a more thorough description of the typical characteristics of each of these somatotypes. After you have determined which body type most closely resembles your own, you can design a workout program to best suit your needs.

The chapter on your body type gives you a clearer idea of what your body type is, which characteristics you got from your parents, and which ones you may pass on if you have kids. Chapter 8 guides you through a fitness evaluation process and helps you set up your personalized workout program.

Reasons why exercise is worth the sweat

What are some of your reasons why you can't fit exercise into your lifestyle? I won't buy the lack of time excuse. Everyone has at least 15 minutes a few days a week to get a little physical activity. It doesn't matter whether you do your squats while brushing your teeth or curl your biceps by lifting your child. Just do it. For every reason you can give me why you can't exercise, I can give you a better reason why you should. Here's a challenge for you. Read the list below and then let me know if you still feel a little exercise isn't worth the time.

Exercise can help you:

- Develop a healthy, fit body.
- Control your body weight.
- Maintain good posture.
- Improve your muscles' strength, endurance, and tone.
- Strengthen your joints.
- Increase the flexibility of your joints and muscles.
- Improve your cardiovascular fitness.
- Reduce stress.
- Increase the efficiency of your circulatory and respiratory systems.
- Reduce the risks of cardiovascular disease and stroke.
- Improve your self-esteem.
- Decrease your body fat.
- Increase your muscle mass.
- Control your appetite.
- Improve your sports performance.
- Improve your work performance.
- Increase the efficiency of your digestive system.
- Decrease your risk of injury.
- Improve your mental awareness.
- Improve your self-confidence.
- Sleep soundly.
- Increase your energy.
- Improve your rate of metabolism.
- Lengthen your life span.

Remember: One key to getting in shape or just staying fit and healthy is to be consistent. Whether you have a formal exercise regime or are starting out by increasing your physical activity during your daily life, your goal should be to stick with it. The amount of time you spend working out isn't nearly as important as exercising consistently. Your results, of course, depend to a great extent on the length and intensity of your workouts, but the important part is to form a habit. If you can maintain consistency, increasing the intensity comes much more easily.

Chapter 2

The "Where" and "Wear" of Working Out: Shoes, Clothes, and More

- -

- -

Many people have a favorite room in their home that they enjoy relaxing in or just like to hang out in. The same goes for clothing. Have you ever noticed if you have a few particular outfits that are really comfortable and that seem to be a regular part of your wardrobe? My favorite comfy clothes would have to be my sweatshirt and sweatpants! Generally, fitness clothing should be comfortable, loose-fitting, and made of cotton or a breathable material. Having an environment that you feel comfortable in and clothes that make you feel good are an important part of getting yourself motivated to work out. If you've chosen to do your workout in your home, find a place you enjoy being in, but make sure it provides you with the space you need to move around without knocking over anything breakable or injuring yourself on a coffee table. Placing a mirror in the room can help you pay attention to your form as you exercise or just admire yourself, and good ventilation and a fan can keep you going when you start to work up a sweat. If you choose to work out outside, make sure it's not too hot or humid. I prefer to find a nice shady spot or work out early in the morning before the sun gets too hot. Throw on some clothes that are comfortable and put on a pair of workout shoes to suit your exercise. If you're comfortable and feel good about your environment, you'll enjoy your workouts that much more.

Give Me My Space

How much space do you need for a workout? It really depends on what you plan to do in your workout. Based on an average person's size and the exercises I list in this book, an adequate space should probably be at least 6 feet by 8 feet (1.8 meters by 2.4 meters). This measurement doesn't mean that you can't do the same exercises in a more confined area. If you plan on doing the muscle conditioning exercises in this book, take a moment to scout out your workout area.

- ✔ Make sure your workout area is free of things you can trip over, like cords, or things you can fall into, like your television.

- ✔ Determine how much space you need by standing in the center point of your workout area and lunging forward, backward, and to both sides. If you have enough room to comfortably move about, you're ready to work out.

Choosing an Indoor Floor Surface

At home you are limited to what types of floor surfaces you can work out on. Most of us have carpet, tile, linoleum or wood floors. Depending on what you plan to do or what type of activity you'll be doing on the surface, there are a few key things to look at before you begin.

Whenever you're performing exercises that require twisting or a quick change in direction, a flat surface like wood or tile flooring is best. Carpet can catch your shoe and make turning moves more difficult. This type of movement on a carpeted surface can place undue stress on the joints in your knee.

If you plan to jump, dance or do any type of low- to high-impact aerobic moves, you want to make sure your floor surface will absorb the impact. This means your concrete basement floor should not be your first choice location to practice jumping rope. In this case, it's best to find a floor that has some sort of padding to absorb the shock of your movements. Even if you don't have a carpeted floor, many linoleum and wood floors have underlying shock absorption.

If you're doing the muscle-conditioning exercises in this book, however, a carpet or other soft, flat surface works just fine. If you're working out on a hard surface, it's best to have an exercise mat to lie on while doing floor exercises. You can find a wide variety of inexpensive mats in sporting goods stores.

Overall, look for a non-slip surface to work out on. If you choose to work out on wood, tile, or linoleum, make sure you don't slip on sweat that drips onto the floor. Carpet is good for stepping or muscle-conditioning exercises because it provides good traction and a padded surface. Concrete is the worst choice and should be avoided, if possible.

Keep in mind that a floor surface alone can't prevent injuries — an appropriate shoe, safe exercises, and a floor that absorbs some of the impact on your body is a good combination to work with.

A Shoe for Every Activity

Don't run or walk in old, worn-out shoes, or the ones that your dog used as a chew toy. They provide little or no support and can increase your chances of getting injured. Try to wear your workout shoes only when you're exercising, not when you go to the beach, go shopping, or walk around the house. Keep a separate pair of walking shoes for daily activities.

After you choose the types of exercise you plan to participate in, look for shoes that are designed specifically for that sport or activity and the movements it requires. For example, running involves a forward movement in which your foot contacts the ground in a heel to toe motion. Because of the impact on your joints during running, shoe cushioning is critical. Tennis, on the other hand, requires a shoe with more lateral support (movements that require a side to side motion). Before you run out to purchase a new pair of shoes, take a moment to learn what to look for in a fitness shoe.

What to look for in a shoe

Thanks to the many footwear companies, you have a variety of quality shoes to choose from. The most important factor is comfort; having proper fit enhances your workout and lowers any possibility of foot injury. Wearing a shoe that gives you no support or is uncomfortable to wear can lead to ankle injury and add stress to bones and joints in your foot, lower leg, knee, and hip. Depending on the impact of the exercise, some shock waves can travel up to the lower spine and cause discomfort to back muscles. So begin with comfort and support and then select a shoe for the appropriate sport or activity. You have four key elements to look for in a shoe:

- ✔ Shock absorption
- ✔ Fit
- ✔ Flexibility
- ✔ Stability

Absorbing the SHOCK

Shock absorption is one of the most important reasons to wear and buy a sport or activity shoe. Without shock absorption, your feet not only take a pounding, you increase the risk of injury to your feet, legs, knees, and lower back. Most shoes have a three-layer sole where cushioning is dispersed among an outer, mid, and inner sole.

The *outer sole* is made with the most durable material — rubber, which can withstand the initial impact, grip, and traction. Certain designs in the rubber of the outer sole are called *flex grooves* and can help prevent blisters and fatigue.

The *mid sole* is where most of the shock absorbency is received. Depending on the activity the shoe is designed for, extra shock absorbing material like nitrogen, air, or gel is placed in the heel counter of the shoe. Keep in mind that shoes lose their cushioning and absorption after about three months of consistent use.

Last, an *inner sole* is located above the mid-sole and may add extra arch support or act like an orthotic insert. This is good news for stinky feet because you can take out inner soles and wash them.

Finding the right FIT for your footprint

Just as you have a certain body type, you also have a special foot design. Whether you have a flat foot, curved foot, arched foot, or fat foot, each requires a certain type of footwear. Before you purchase shoes, it's good to know what type of foot you have so you can find a shoe that suits your needs.

Take a look at your feet. Stand up straight and have someone look at your feet from the instep (the inside of your feet). This can get personal, so find someone who won't be offended by your feet. If your partner can place a middle finger between the arch of your foot and the floor you have a *high arch;* if not, you have a *flat foot.* Next, have your partner stand behind you and see if your foot rolls slightly outward or inward from the ankle as you walk.

Another way to check this is by looking at your shoes to see where they are worn out. If you see that they are worn on the outer side of the heel you have a *supinated* foot. A curved foot with a high arch is known as a supinated foot, and it allows the foot to roll outward as you walk. This supination can put pressure on the outer structure of the foot and travel upward toward the side of your knee and hip joint. A shoe with medial (middle) arch support is needed for this type of foot. The opposite of supination is *pronation,* which is evident when the instep of a shoe is the first place to wear out. This happens to a foot that is flat and appears to lean inward at the ankle and knee joint. This type of foot needs a shoe with good arch support in the mid-sole of the shoe.

Having FLEXIBILITY

It's the flexibility of a shoe that gives your foot the freedom to move. A special material called multidensity polymer is used in the mid-sole of the shoe (between the shock absorption layer and the outermost sole) to allow your foot to bend easily and provide the flexibility feature to your fitness shoes. Here is an easy way to check a new shoe's flexibility. Hold the shoe in your hand and bend the toe box to the heel. If the shoe feels stiff in the mid sole, it's probably too thick — and this may cause a muscle imbalance, shin splints, and pain in your lower extremities. If you find that you can easily twist the shoe from side to side, this shoe probably has too much flexibility for side to side movements like the ones performed in aerobic dance, basketball, or tennis.

Staying STABLE

The type of activity you plan on participating in determines the type of stability you need to look for in your shoes. Here are a few examples. The makeup of a good dance aerobic shoe and court shoe allows for lateral or side to side motion, high- and/or low-impact movements, and turns. You don't want your foot rolling over from side to side, so look for external support straps across the forefoot to give you extra stability. If a running shoe is what you're after, look for support in the heel to hold the rear of your foot in place as you jog or run. If step aerobics is your choice of cardiovascular activity, look for a step shoe with all-around stability both in the rear and forefoot. Some shoes are designed with a high top or mid cut for extra support around your ankles. Just make sure the material around your ankle is not too stiff and is made of an ultra-light material.

The following lists show you some things to look for when buying athletic shoes and the most popular shoes being sold for each activity.

Running and jogging comfortably

Injuries to your knees, joints, or back are always a risk when you participate in high-impact activities like jogging and running. To keep yourself safe, look for a breathable, lightweight shoe that offers cushioning in the heel and forefoot. If you *pronate* your feet when your run (roll your foot toward the center of your body), look for a shoe with a stabilizing device. Your best bet is to shop in an athletic shoe store and ask a knowledgeable salesperson to fit you for a shoe based on your stride, instep, and foot arch needs. See Table 2-1 for suggestions.

Table 2-1	Suggested Running and Jogging Shoes
Women	*Men*
Saucony	Asics
Asics	Nike
Brooks	New Balance
	Adidas

Finding cushy aerobic shoes

An aerobic shoe is a good choice for an all-encompassing gym shoe. Look for cushion in the forefoot and lots of lateral support for those side-to-side steps. You'll find these shoes in low top or mid cut. Make your choice based on your ankle comfort and the support the shoe provides. Check out Table 2-2 for top aerobic shoe picks.

Table 2-2	Great Aerobic Shoes
Women	*Men*
Avia	Nike court or cross-training shoes
Ryka	Reebok court or cross-training shoes
Reebok	
Nike	

Walking your way to comfort

Flexibility and stability are key points to remember when purchasing your walking shoes. You need flexibility in the forefoot to allow for natural movement and stability in the heel of the shoe. A good walking shoe has a slight dome (curve or angle) in the heel for extra support. Table 2-3 lists some of my recommendations for walking shoes.

Table 2-3	Recommended Walking Shoes
Women	*Men*
New Balance	New Balance
Reebok	Reebok
Nike	Rockport

Cross training in comfort

With a name like "cross trainer" you may think that these shoes are the answer to the perfect all-sport shoe. Although the cross trainer is suitable for many activities, it's always preferable to put your best foot forward in a shoe designed for the activity you plan to participate in. The good thing about these shoes is that they lighten up your gym bag and keep your wallet full. Cross trainers are made with good ankle support, good lateral movement stability, and enhanced shock absorption. These shoes are best used for aerobic dance, weight training, step aerobics, and walking. See Table 2-4 for help in picking out cross trainers.

Table 2-4	Choosing Cross Trainers
Women	*Men*
Asics	New Balance
New Balance	Reebok
Ryka	

Bicycling footwear

Although you can wear a versatile cross training shoe to walk on the treadmill or jump around in a step aerobics class, you can't throw on your cycling shoes for any other activity other than bicycling. Cycling shoes are made with clips on the bottom and are designed specifically for both stationary and road bikes. Don't try stepping in these shoes unless you're looking for a broken neck.

If you plan on attending spinning classes, which is a group class where each student has his or her own stationary bike and follows the teacher's lead, look for a shoe that has good ventilation, a stiff sole, and adjustable closure straps. The pedals of road bikes and the bikes designed for spinning classes require shoes with toe clips. There are currently two types: *Look* or *SPD* shoe clips. The SPD stands for Shimano Peddling Dynamics, which is the company that manufactures this toe clip. It is smaller than the Look clip and easier to walk on, but also more expensive. The Look toe clip is a bit larger and fills up more surface area which makes it easier to slide your foot onto. This clip is used more by road cyclists. Ask your cycling teacher to advise you on which clip or shoe works best with the bikes for the class. If you want to be able to get off your bike and actually walk around, the shoes to purchase are the ones made for mountain biking (Look toe clips). The clip on these shoes is recessed in the sole of the shoes, enabling you to walk around.

What to Wear When You Work Out

In my aerobics classes, I always see the students in the front row with the latest fashion trends in fitness. These are the men and women who are looking good, know all the moves, and want to be noticed. Why not? They work hard to make their bodies fit. The back row is a different story. Usually, people in the back row wear big, oversized T-shirts and sweats, and look as if they can't wait for the class to end. Over a period of time, however, and with consistent workouts, they too move up a few rows and start sporting the newest aerobic fashions as their muscles bloom and their confidence increases. Don't get me wrong — working out in style is fine, but the most important aspect of this story is the increase in confidence — something you should strive for.

Here are some things to consider when selecting fitness clothing to wear for your workout.

- ✔ What time of day are you exercising?
- ✔ Are you exercising inside or outside?
- ✔ What are the weather and temperature like outside?
- ✔ What type of activity are you doing?
- ✔ Which body parts do you want to show off?
- ✔ Which body parts do you want to hide?

Your first priority when choosing your workout wear is comfort. Weather conditions are your most important concern if you plan on exercising outdoors. You may remember your parents layering clothes on you when you went out to play during the winter months. You may have looked like a big goofy snowman, but you were probably warm. Dressing in layers allows you the option of removing or adding clothes depending on your body temperature. In addition, you can limit the amount of body heat you lose from your head and hands by wearing a hat and gloves while exercising in cool climates.

Have you ever gone white-water rafting? One thing they ask you NOT to wear is cotton. You're sure to get wet and cotton only makes you stay wet, cold, and feel heavy. Cotton absorbs moisture and clings to your skin, making you feel weighted down. If you're in a cold climate or are guaranteed to get soaked when you work out, you want to have fabrics that absorb moisture and sweat but then whisk it away from your body. Supplex is one of my favorite fabrics for workout wear because it not only absorbs moisture, it breathes, is flexible, and its colors don't fade. Your clothes look newer longer and wear better.

Exercising in warm weather requires lighter clothing that allows you to move easily. Cotton, due to its ability to absorb sweat, is a good choice for exercise clothes for warm-weather workouts. Don't forget your sweatbands for the head and wrists. If you're a "sweater" like some of my friends are (I won't mention their names), you may find that a headband can help prevent sweat from rushing into your eyes. A sweatband on your wrist can be used to wipe beads of perspiration off just about anywhere on your body. Remember: If you're comfortable with what you're wearing (and you're having fun doing a particular activity), you'll stick with it a lot longer and see the results of your hard work sooner.

If you're trying to pack on the muscle, you're going to spend some time with weights in your hands. Unless you like the look of calluses, you need to wear gloves. The gloves, which are made out of Neoprene (a material used to make wetsuits), have a tendency to deteriorate easily. I've found that bicycle gloves hold up the best. Find a glove made from a natural material that covers your knuckles and the top portion of your fingers. They should fit firmly (you know, "like a glove") but not too tightly.

Aside from keeping warm and dry during your workout, you may want to wear clothes that flatter your figure. Fitness clothing manufacturers have helped to establish the trend in workout wear. Aerobic clothes and clothes made specifically for runners and cyclists can be found in most department stores, however, the tried and true T-shirt and gym shorts still prevail in most gyms around America. More important than your wardrobe is keeping your body hydrated. Don't forget your water bottle. Drink before, during, and after your workouts.

The do's and don'ts of workout clothes

If you're looking for workout clothes that conceal flaws in your figure, take a look at the do's and don'ts:

✔ Don't wear tight tank tops if you're self-conscious of your chest or carry extra weight in your upper body.

✔ Don't wear cutoff shirts or pants with a tight waist if you are heavy around the mid-section.

✔ Do wear shorts or pants with an adjustable elastic waistband to lessen bulging around the waistline.

✔ Don't wear shorts or pants with horizontal stripes or loud prints, especially flowers, if you have a butt you're trying to hide.

✔ Do wear dark-colored bottoms to slenderize your bottom half.

✔ Don't wear short shorts if your thighs move back and forth faster than your feet do.

✔ Do wear shorter length bottoms if you want your legs to look longer.

Chapter 3

Warming Up, Cooling Down, and Stretching

*I*f you didn't have to warm up and stretch before your workout, then cool down and stretch after your workout, you could cut at least 10 or 15 minutes from your total exercise time. Some of you have surely thought about this when you're feeling a little short on time. Maybe you jumped out of bed in the morning, threw on your running shoes, and headed for the hills without time to warm up or stretch your waking muscles. You may get by without much discomfort later that day or even the next, but over time you'll begin to injure your joints, causing premature arthritis. As you get older, jumping into your workout becomes more difficult, because your body needs a bit more time to get in gear. Warming up and cooling down can help you ease your way into and out of your workout.

Whether you're in top physical condition or attempting to get into shape, the best ways to prevent unnecessary muscle soreness or injury are to dedicate a small portion of your workout to warming up your muscles, stretching your body, and cooling down for a few minutes after you work out.

Why Your Body Needs to Warm Up and Cool Down

You should warm up before a strenuous workout or activity to prepare your body for more vigorous exercise. By beginning your workout with a warm-up, you elevate your body temperature and heart rate, loosen up your joints, and get the blood flowing to your muscles. When you are finished with your workout, a cool down period allows your body and cardiovascular system to slow down and gradually recover.

Warming up your engine before you speed up

When you're getting ready to drive your car, you usually allow it to warm up before you take off. Why shouldn't you do the same for your body? Warming up your car's engine prepares it for rushing through the morning traffic and picking up speed on the highway. Just like your car, your body needs preparation in order to go from a resting state to active motion. You don't jump out of bed, sprint to the toilet (unless you really have to go), run to the kitchen, and chug your coffee, do you? Going from 0 to 100 miles per hour isn't the safest way to start your day *or* to start exercising.

The following list shows you a few ways you can benefit from your warm-ups:

- Your muscle metabolism is more efficient at slightly higher temperatures (and your body temperature rises as you begin to warm up).
- Warm-ups may help to prevent injury during your workout.
- You increase the blood flow to your heart and muscles.
- You increase the flexibility of your joint and connective tissues.
- The lubrication within your joints is increased, making it easier for you to move your limbs.

Cooling down, not falling down

At the end of your workout (especially vigorous cardiovascular exercise), you need to give your body time to recover and allow your heart rate to fall back down to 120 beats per minute or less (see Chapter 10 for heart rate charts). Reserving time to cool your body down helps maintain the blood flow to your heart, which can prevent a cardiac disturbance. As a safety precaution you should allow your heart rate and the flow of blood to and from your heart to decrease gradually. After a hard cardiovascular workout you can slow down your heart rate by doing the same activity you just did, but at a much slower pace. You can also simply walk around for a few minutes. Whichever you choose, don't just stop and drop to the ground. This can cause painful muscle contractions and pooling of the blood in your lower extremities.

Have you ever watched horses race? In readiness for the race, jockeys and the horses are led around the track. The horses maintain a light gallop, which prepares their muscles and joints to run. The jockeys mimic their riding positions in order to prepare for the ride. At the end of the race, the horses don't simply stop; they slow down and gallop lightly again. This allows them to cool down by relaxing their muscles and slowing down their heart rates and cardiovascular systems.

 The more fit you are, the faster you recover. Fit people can restore their bodies to their normal resting state faster than deconditioned individuals because they have better control of temperature and blood flow, and better stress hormone regulation.

If you're just starting to exercise, you may notice that throughout your cool-down your heart is still racing and you're huffin' and puffin' like a dragon. If you consistently work out, this changes, and your recovery time will be dramatically reduced. For example, if you have been running consistently for many years, your heart rate recovery time may only take a few minutes, whereas if you've just begun to run for exercise, your recovery period may take 10 minutes or more. You can track your recovery time by checking your heart rate one minute after you finish exercising (see Chapter 10 for heart rate charts). As you become more physically fit, your heart rate returns to its normal beat more quickly than when you first began exercising.

Choosing a Warm-Up and a Cool-Down

You can create your own warm-up or pick one from one of the following. If you're not feeling extremely coordinated, your best bet is to warm up your body by mimicking your planned workout.

Mimic warm-up

 Mimic the workout you're preparing for, but do it without any resistance, or at a low level of intensity. Make sure you move your body through a full *range of motion* (ROM). This means you can't be sluggish in your warm-up movements. When you move your arms and legs through their full range of motion, you are moving them to their full extent in both directions. If I asked you to swing your arms up and down through their full range of motion, if you had the ability, you would swing your arms up over your head, then back down to your legs. You know the range in which your body feels comfortable, so make the most out of your warm-up and complete each movement.

For an example of a warm-up that mimics your intended workout, you can prepare to run on the treadmill by spending the first three minutes walking at a comfortable pace. Before you play tennis, you may want to spend a few minutes walking briskly and jogging around the court, practice swinging your racket through a full range of motion without hitting a ball, and then try hitting a few backhands, forehands, and serves. When you're weight training, you can get blood flowing through your muscles if you ride the stationary bike for 5 minutes, then run through the motions of your weight lifting routine without using any resistance. As you perform your muscle conditioning exercises, you can do a few repetitions using light resistance to better prepare your body.

Move your feet warm-up

If you live in a two-story home you can warm up for your workout by simply walking up and down the stairs for about five minutes, which initiates an increase in your heart rate. If you're like me and live in a one-story home, try the following warm-up to get your feet moving.

1. **March in place and alternate swinging your arms forward and back.**

2. **Alternate lifting your knees toward your chest. Starting with your arms over your head, pull one hand down to touch your opposite knee and then alternate each hand to the opposite knee.**

3. **Change your knee lifts to alternate kicks forward, reaching your hands toward your feet.**

4. **Swing your arms from side to side, moving your body in the same direction as your arms.**

5. **Repeat from the top.**

Swing and reach warm-up

Have you ever seen people strutting their stuff on the dance floor, looking like they're mimicking their aerobic dance classes? Well, they probably are. Whether you like to dance before you work out, or just do a little swinging and reaching, you'll find this warm-up simple and effective.

1. **Start swinging both arms alternately forward and backward, and then swing them together. Add a small squat by bending your knees slightly. As your arms come forward, extend your knees and lift yourself onto your toes.**

2. Stand with both feet shoulder width apart and reach your right arm over your head and diagonally across to the left side of your head. Continue by alternating your arms from right to left.

3. Raise both arms up from the sides of your body until they reach shoulder level. Now alternate reaching each arm out side to side. Keep your hips still and allow your upper body to move with your arms.

4. Roll your shoulders forward (toward your neck) 8 times, then roll them backward 8 times.

5. Repeat from the top.

Cooling down

Cooling down can include the same activities you used to warm up. Depending on how strenuous your workouts are, you may need to spend only 5 to 10 minutes cooling down. The main thing is to keep moving and gradually decrease the intensity of your exercise. Give yourself a chance to relax and let your body temperature decrease naturally before you jump into a hot shower or a hot tub. Breathing is also important. As you slow down the intensity of your workout, try to slow down your breathing. Take long, deep breaths and concentrate on inhaling and exhaling from your diaphragm (belly region). Avoid short, shallow breathing from your chest (see "Tips for daily breathing" later in this chapter). As long as you give your body time to slow down, while keeping it moving, you're good to go. Have fun and make up your own warm-ups and cool-downs.

Warm-up and cool-down do's and don'ts

✔ Do give yourself 3 to 10 minutes to warm up before you work out.

✔ Do move your joints through a full range of motion during your warm-up.

✔ Do allow your heart and muscles 2 to 5 minutes to cool down and recover from your workout.

✔ Do perform both your warm-up and cool-down at a lower intensity than your workout, and without much resistance.

✔ Do start out easy, move slowly, and build up your speed gradually.

✔ Do breathe throughout your warm-up, stretch, and cool-down. (Just a reminder in case you were planning on holding your breath.)

✔ Do listen to your body. If you feel pain, back off, slow down, or stop the movement.

✔ Don't stop and sit down after a cardiovascular workout; walk it out.

✔ Don't skip your warm-up because you think you don't have time.

Increasing Your Flexibility

Can you bend over and touch your toes? If you find your fingers are dangling above your knees as you reach for your toes, you better start stretching. Many factors affect flexibility, including age, gender, body type, and level of activity. As you age, your joints lose flexibility, especially if you've been sedentary most of your life. In order for your joints to stay in shape, you need to use them for their purposes: flexion and extension.

In regard to gender, women are generally more flexible than men. But your body type (see Chapters 5 through 7 to determine yours) may also be a determining factor in flexibility. For example, if you're an ectomorph, (check out Chapter 6), you tend to have longer, leaner muscles that allow you a greater range of flexibility than a mesomorph, (described in Chapter 5), who may have bigger, bulkier muscles.

Finally, the more sedentary your lifestyle is, the less flexible you are. If your daily exercise is getting up and down from the couch, chances are you need to stretch. Muscles that aren't stretched become shorter and tighter. Instead of sitting on the couch when you're watching television, sit on the floor and do a few stretches while you watch your favorite show. Any way you look at it, muscle and joint flexibility is just as important as good cardiovascular and muscle conditioning workout programs.

The Benefits of Stretching

After sleeping, your muscles need to stretch before they're able to reach their full range of motion. (They naturally tighten up while at rest.) Also, your body temperature is low, and muscles should be warm before you begin your stretch, so try to avoid jumping out of bed and into your favorite yoga position. In the same way a rubber band stretches to a certain range before returning to its starting point, your muscles should be lengthened during a stretch and then relaxed. By stretching regularly you can increase the flexibility and elasticity of your muscles, loosen up your joints, improve your posture, and improve your ability to perform in sports and daily activities.

Stretching reduces the risk of soreness in your muscles

After a workout, it's best to stretch the muscles you used while exercising. Some researchers have found that by stretching your muscles after you work out, you can decrease the amount of muscle soreness you may experience in the following days. If you do have a great deal of muscle soreness after your workout, take caution and continue to stretch *gently*.

Tips for daily breathing

Breathing is a key element during stretching and other activities like yoga, pilates, or weight training. By breathing correctly, you help your muscles relax and lessen the tension on your ligaments during a stretch or muscle contraction. If you've ever been frightened when you had to speak in public, you may have noticed the tension in your body and the tightness of your muscles. The best advice probably came from someone who told you to breathe deeply and slowly in order to calm and relax yourself. Use that advice in your everyday life and you'll begin to feel better all over.

✔ **Breathing from your diaphragm:** Lie on your back and place your hands on your abdomen. Notice how your belly expands and relaxes with each breath you take. When your abdominal muscles are relaxed, you allow your diaphragm to fully expand and contract with each breath. Your chest, on the other hand, hardly moves as you breathe. Now stand up and do the same thing. Try to concentrate on seeing your diaphragm (located underneath your belly) expanding and contracting naturally, and keep your chest as still as possible.

✔ **Breathing deep to de-stress:** Close your eyes (as long as you're not driving) and listen to your breath. Listen to it entering and exiting your body with each inhale and exhale. Now, find an area of tension in your body. As you inhale, imagine yourself breathing into that specific spot. Breathe deeply, expanding your diaphragm. As you slowly release your breath, let go of the tension and relax. Ah!

✔ **Breathing while stretching:** First and most importantly: *Don't hold your breath.* As you inhale, your body takes in oxygen that penetrates the blood being sent to your muscles. If you hold your breath, you're depriving yourself of this oxygenated blood. Breathe deeply and slowly throughout your stretch. Inhale deeply as you begin your stretch, and slowly release your breath as you follow through the movement. Continue to breathe deeply as you hold the stretch.

Note: If you want to learn more about breathing techniques, check out *Conscious Breathing: Breathwork for health, stress release, and personal mastery,* by Gay Hendricks, Ph.D., published in 1997 by Bantam Books.

Stretching reduces your risk of injury

The last thing you, as an active person, want is an injury that keeps you from working out, especially if you make a living from having a healthy, strong body. Even if your body is not the means of your income (and don't take that the wrong way), you can prevent everyday injuries if you have flexible muscles and joints. Let's say, for instance, that you're a weekend workout warrior and you played hard on Sunday afternoon, but neglected to stretch. Monday morning comes along, and as you attempt to get out of bed, you pull your hamstring muscles because they're tight from yesterday's activities. The tension in your hamstrings causes you back pain (because these sets of muscles are connected to each other) and your joints are sore. Next thing you know, you miss your workout and maybe even your job for a day or two. You may think I sound like your mother, but if you've had this happen to you before, you know why I'm warning you.

Stretching can help you to relax both mentally and physically

The fewer times your body feels stress, the more it can relax. The stress your muscles receive during your workout is good, but on the other hand, the stress your body receives when you have a bad day at work or home can cause both physical and mental tension. By implementing a consistent stretch routine in your daily life and learning to breathe correctly (see the sidebar "Tips for daily breathing" and the section "Stretching Your Options" later in this chapter for help), you can relax your body and clear your mind.

TAMILEE SAYS

Stretching in the sky

Stretching has benefited me innumerable times. One in particular was a return flight from Japan to Los Angeles, which was approximately ten hours. This flight made me realize the benefits of being short. I could stretch my legs straight out to the seat in front of me, so every time the guy in front of me got up, I put my feet up on his seat and gave myself a hamstring stretch. I tried to drink eight ounces of water every hour, which sent me to the bathroom several times. Each time I took a few moments to stretch my legs, back, and upper body. While I sat in my little seat, I tried to work on deep-relaxation breathing techniques. At times I noticed people looking over at me as if I were a weirdo, but after a while I saw a few of them stretching their necks and shoulders and doing some deep breathing. Though the flight was a drag due to the duration, from that time on I've made stretch breaks on the plane an important part of my travel routine.

Stretching can help you feel better all over

As you age, not only do your muscles lose elasticity, but your bones get brittle and your tendons and ligaments become more susceptible to injury. Stretching lengthens your muscles, which helps them to maintain their elasticity. In the long run, you'll look and feel better.

Stretching Your Options

Stretching is not only good for you but also helps you to feel good. Whether you are loosening up for a night of dancing or just relaxing after a stressful day, stretching can reenergize your body and mind. Several types or styles of stretching have been developed over the years. Try each one and see which is most comfortable and beneficial to you.

Static stretching

Though many different methods of stretching exist, the most common method is *static stretching,* which involves the use of a position held for a particular period of time. Try a static stretch on your hamstring muscle, for example. Sit on the floor with your legs extended in front of you, and then slowly lower your upper body toward your legs. Feel the pull, or stretch, in your hamstrings, gluteus muscles, and back. Remember to stretch until you feel tightness, not pain, and hold your position for a period of 10 to 30 seconds. Research studies have noted that static stretching is the preferred and safer method of stretching because it produces less muscle soreness and less energy expenditure than other types and can provide muscles with relief from tension and stress.

Ballistic stretching

An alternate form of stretching, predominately used by dancers, is *ballistic stretching.* Ballistic stretching is defined as bouncing, bobbing, or rhythmic motion. One of the major arguments against this type of stretch technique is that it increases the risk of soreness to the muscle, pulling a muscle, or injuring the muscle tissue. If the tissue or muscle is stretched too rapidly, you may not develop optimal flexibility. Instead of relaxing the muscle, the quick reflex action of the stretched muscle causes it to contract. This increases muscle tension and makes it more difficult to stretch out the connective tissue and more likely that you risk injury. In general, ballistic stretching is not recommended as a warm-up exercise.

Passive stretching

Passive stretching is yet another way to increase your flexibility. You need a partner or outside force (like a towel or piece of equipment) to perform this type of stretch. This form of stretching is most frequently used by physical therapists or personal trainers. The main purpose of passive stretching is to lengthen the elastic portion of your muscle. This is done passively to restore the normal range of motion to a joint or muscle that has lost a substantial amount of soft tissue. If you want to try this type of stretch without a partner, do the following calf stretch. Grab a towel and sit on the floor with your feet out in front of you. Place the towel under one foot and hang on to each end of the towel with one hand. Keep this leg flat on the floor with your heel down and your toes pointed up toward the ceiling. Begin to stretch your calf by pulling the ends of the towel toward the mid-section of your body. Do not resist the force of the towel — just allow it to pull the ball of your foot toward you. Hold this position for 10 to 30 seconds and then release it. This stretch can, of course, be done with a partner or personal trainer. Instead of a towel, your partner uses his or her hands to passively create the stretch in your muscle.

Passive active stretching

The *passive active* stretch is similar to passive stretching because it uses an outside force to assist you in stretching a muscle. The difference is that you attempt to hold the stretch by contracting your muscle isometrically for a few seconds (contracting your muscle against an immovable force). This type of stretch can help strengthen the muscle opposite of the muscle you are stretching. For example, if you are stretching your hamstring muscles, you simultaneously strengthen your quadricep muscles, which is the opposing muscle group to the hamstrings. To demonstrate this style of stretch, look to the example of the calf stretch in the previous section. The only difference between the two styles is that you are more active or aggressive in this type of stretch. You resist the towel or your partner who is creating the stretch on your calf muscle. By simultaneously contracting your calf as it is being stretched, you increase your flexibility as well as slightly strengthen the opposing muscle, which is your tibia.

Proprioceptive Neuromuscular Facilitation (PNF) stretching

Use this term at the next cocktail party you attend and you'll impress all your friends. I love to demonstrate PNF stretching at my workshops, because you can see instant results. This method entails stimulation of the neuromuscular mechanism by proprioceptors, which are little organs that hang out in your tendons. They monitor tension and stretch, then send feedback to your brain. Your muscle is stretched to the point of limitation in a PNF technique. One method of using this technique is to isometrically contract the muscle *prior* to an extensive stretch, then continue by stretching the muscle until it has reached its limitation, and hold it for approximately 10 seconds. (Remember: An isometric stretch is a stretch against an immovable force.) This series can be repeated a few times to extend the stretch even further. When the contraction is released, the muscle you stretched is able to increase its range of motion and has the capacity to stretch further. Just like magic, right? The truth is that the proprioceptors are stimulated, giving the muscle the ability to stretch a little further. This method is usually used by physical therapists because it produces the largest gains in flexibility.

How Long Should You Stretch?

How long you hold a stretch depends on your fitness level. If you are deconditioned, (see Chapter 10 for an assessment), try stretching at least 3 times a week for 20 to 30 minutes each time, holding each stretch for 10 to 30 seconds.

Stretching do's and don'ts

While you are stretching, don't forget the following:

✔ Do make sure you stretch your muscles when they are warm, not cold (after your warm-up or workout).

✔ Do breathe deeply all the way through each stretch.

✔ Do listen to your body and know how far to push yourself.

Mild tension during a stretch is normal, but do not go beyond the point where you experience pain. Besides an inability to go any farther in your stretch, another indication of your limit is when your muscle shakes as it reaches the point of tightness.

Think of it as your muscle saying, "That's enough — don't go any farther!" At this point you should stop, hold the stretch where it is most comfortable for you, and take a few deep breaths before you release the stretch.

✔ Do hold each stretch for at least 10 seconds. (But holding a stretch for more than 30 seconds doesn't provide any additional benefit.)

✔ Don't bounce.

✔ Don't lock your joints.

Remember that increasing your flexibility takes time. Be patient — good things come in time.

If you're already in the habit of exercising, give your body a stretch at the end of each workout (after your cool down). Better yet, try to implement a stretch routine into your schedule 5 times a week for 20 to 30 minutes, holding each stretch for 10 to 30 seconds.

Starting a Stretch Routine

This stretch routine targets muscles from your whole body. You can select a few stretches to do after your workout, or put them all together for a full body stretch regimen.

Quadriceps

Your quads are located on your front upper thigh and are the largest group of muscles in your body. These muscles are at work for you whether you're simply standing up or running a marathon, so regular stretching keeps you limber and improves your performance. Figure 3-1 shows you how to stretch your quadriceps — a good idea before and after exercising. All you need is a chair!

1. **Stand with your back facing the side of a chair.**
2. **Place one foot behind you, with your toes on the seat of the chair.**

   Keep the knee of your standing leg slightly bent and hold onto the back of the chair for balance.
3. **Tighten your gluteus muscle (or bun) of the leg resting on the chair and concentrate on stretching the front of the thigh (quadriceps).**
4. **Hold the stretch and repeat, using your other leg.**

Hamstrings

The hamstring muscles are found in the back of your upper thigh and are the opposing muscle group to your quadriceps. Because the quads are generally stronger than the hamstrings, it is important to stretch the back thigh area to prevent excessive tightness. Tight hamstrings are also the culprits in the cause of low back pain. The correct form for the hamstring stretch is shown in Figure 3-2. But be careful! Pressing on your knee to extend the stretch will cause you to hyperextend the joint in your knee and can cause injury.

1. **Stand facing the side of a chair.**
2. **Place one foot on the seat and keep that leg straight.**

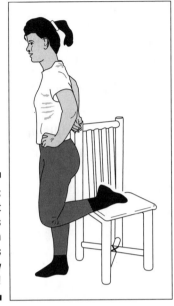

Figure 3-1:
Contract
your buns
to stretch
your quads
— how
easy!

3. **Slowly bend forward from the hips. Place one hand on the chair for balance, and rest your other hand on the opposite thigh (do *not* press down on your knee that is in the stretched position).**

   Feel the stretch to your upper back thigh muscle (hamstrings).

4. **Hold the stretch and repeat, using your other leg.**

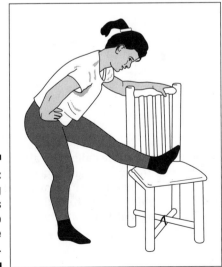

Figure 3-2:
Hamstring
stretches
can help
alleviate
back pain.

Adductors

Figure 3-3 shows a move that's frequently called a lunge. Rather than lunging forward or back, as in the lunge exercise, this stretch focuses on loosening up your inner thighs (or adductors) by lunging from side to side. As you hold the stretch position, remember to mentally focus on stretching the inner thigh muscles of the leg that is elongated.

1. **Stand with your feet a bit wider than shoulder width apart.**

2. **Lunge toward one side, keeping your toes and knees directed forward and your buns pressed backward.**

   Feel the stretch in the inner thigh area of the leg that is straightened out.

3. **Hold the stretch and repeat, using your other leg.**

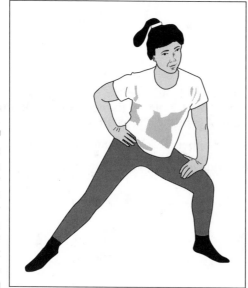

Figure 3-3:
The adductor stretch is a popular move in many workout videos.

Abductors

The outer thigh and hip muscles of your legs are called the abductors. Figure 3-4 demonstrates a great stretch that can be advanced by placing your hand on the knee of your crossed leg and pressing down. Refer to the section on passive stretching earlier in this chapter to find more information on how to enhance this stretch by adding a little resistance to it.

1. **Sit in a chair with one ankle crossed over the opposite knee.**

2. **Slowly bend forward, keeping your crossed leg rotated open (parallel to the ground).**

   You'll feel the stretch in the outer thigh region of your crossed leg.

3. **Hold the stretch and repeat, using your other leg.**

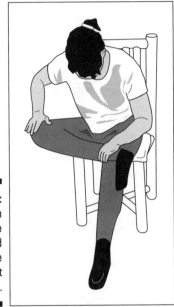

Figure 3-4:
This stretch can be performed anywhere (even at work).

Lower back

Think of putting yourself in the fetal position when doing this stretch. Bringing your knees into your chest, as shown in Figure 3-5, elongates your spine and the muscles of your back. If you have a tendency to sleep on your stomach, or don't have good back support in the chairs you frequently sit in, your muscles become tight from being in a slightly contracted position for a long time. This stretch is perfect in the morning and especially throughout your workday.

1. **Lie on your back with your head and neck relaxed and your knees tucked into your chest.**

2. **The more you pull your legs into your body (keeping your upper back on the floor), the more you feel the stretch in your lower back.**

3. **Hold the stretch and repeat.**

Option: If you are seated in a chair and do not have floor space available, you can do this stretch by bringing your knees toward your chest and tucking your forehead into your knees. It's essentially the same technique, but in a seated position.

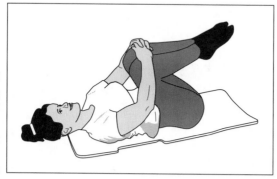

Figure 3-5: This stretch requires a mat or soft surface.

Lats

Lats is the shortened version of latissimus dorsi, which are the muscles that run along the sides of your back. You may already be doing this stretch (shown in Figure 3-6) as you rise and shine in the morning.

1. **Stand with your feet shoulder width apart.**

2. **Clasp your hands together and reach toward the ceiling.**

3. **Slowly bend, flexing your body to one side (not forward or backward).**

   Concentrate on the stretch you feel running along the side of your back down to your waist.

4. **Hold the stretch and repeat on your other side.**

Deltoids

Your deltoids get a bonus, because I list two different stretches. The first version helps stretch the front of your shoulders and the second version stretches the back of your shoulders.

If you've ever spent all day working on a computer or driving a car, you may notice some tightness in the anterior (front) part of your deltoid (shoulder)

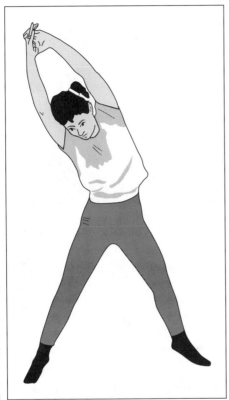

Figure 3-6:
Stretching
your lats
feels great
in the
morning.

muscle. This is usually due to having your arms pulled slightly out in front of you for long periods of time. The stretch in Figure 3-7 puts you in the opposite position to help you loosen up and return to your natural posture.

1. **Stand with your feet shoulder width apart and your hands clasped together behind your back.**

2. **Slowly pull your shoulder blades together and, if possible, elevate your arms toward the ceiling.**

   Feel the stretch in the anterior portion of your deltoid muscle.

3. **Hold the stretch and repeat.**

The second version of the deltoid stretch concentrates on the back of your shoulder muscles. Figure 3-8 shows you a stretch that is very popular among golfers, tennis players, or anyone who tends to overuse the shoulder muscles.

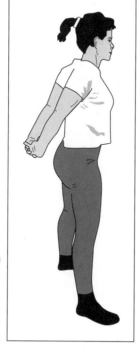

Figure 3-7:
The deltoid
stretch,
version 1.

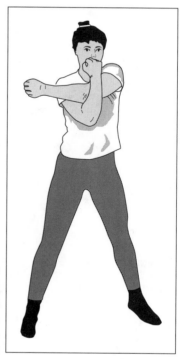

Figure 3-8:
The deltoid
stretch,
version 2.

1. **Stand with your feet shoulder width apart and place one arm across your chest, keeping the elbow of the same arm straight, and its shoulder down.**

2. **With your other hand or arm, pull the straightened arm into your body.**

   This stretch is felt in the posterior (back) portion of your deltoid muscle.

3. **Hold the stretch and repeat it, switching the roles of each arm.**

Biceps

Your bicep muscles, located in the front of your upper arm, are usually in a flexed (slightly bent) position throughout the day, which is why it's important to give them some stretch time. Figure 3-9 offers an easy bicep stretch you can do almost anywhere.

1. **Stand with one arm extended and place your palm on the back of a chair.**

2. **Slowly rotate your body away from the extended arm so that you feel a stretch in the front of your upper arm.**

3. **Hold the stretch and repeat, using your other arm.**

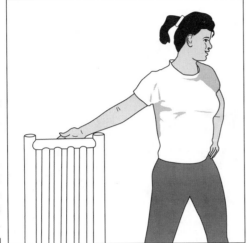

Figure 3-9:
You can also place your palm on a wall for the biceps stretch.

Triceps

One important thing to remember when doing the triceps stretch, shown in Figure 3-10, is to keep your head up and your chin off your chest. By heeding this simple reminder, you'll notice an increase in the stretch of your tricep muscles, which are located in the back of your upper arm.

1. **Sit in a chair with one arm extended overhead.**

2. **Bend the elbow of the extended arm so that you're touching your shoulder (or close to it).**

3. **Carefully (so you don't incur discomfort in your shoulder joint) pull your elbow backward with your other hand.**

   You can feel the stretch in the back of your upper arm.

4. **Hold the stretch and repeat, using your other arm.**

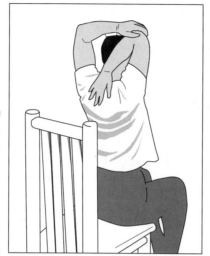

Figure 3-10:
The triceps
stretch
should be
done
carefully to
avoid
discomfort.

Chest

This exercise (shown in Figure 3-11) is one of my favorite stretches, but I've noticed that many people have a tendency to overdo it and end up being sore the next day. The reason for this is because the pectoral (chest) muscles and the joints they are attached to have a greater range of motion to stretch than most muscles.

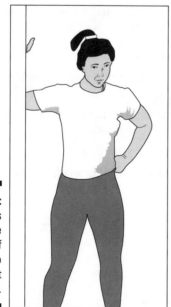

Figure 3-11:
The pecs
have a wide
range of
motion, so
don't
overdo it.

1. **Stand with your forearm against the edge of a wall or doorframe. Raise your elbow so that it's aligned with your shoulder.**

2. **Take a step forward, so that the arm against the wall is now behind you.**

   Stretch your chest muscles (pectorals) only as far as you're comfortable by moving forward an appropriate distance.

3. **Hold the stretch and repeat, using your other arm.**

Upper back

Some people carry a lot of stress and tension in their upper back muscles. The easy stretch shown in Figure 3-12 is a great way to relieve your tension and relax throughout the day.

1. **Sit in a chair with your arms extended in front of your body and your hands clasped together.**

2. **As you reach forward with your arms, round your mid and upper back.**

3. **Drop your chin to your chest and imagine someone pulling your hands away from your body as you resist.**

   This stretch is felt through your upper back and neck.

4. **Hold the stretch and repeat.**

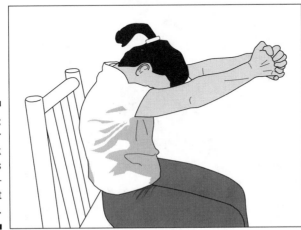

Figure 3-12: The upper back stretch is portable — take it everywhere.

Chapter 4

Listening to Your Body: Injury Prevention

Do you listen to your stomach when it growls, warning you of its hunger and need for food? Do you notice the goose bumps that pop up on your skin when you're cold? You probably acknowledge these signs from your body and respond by taking care of its needs. So why would you ignore your body when it gives a signal like, "Hey, enough already. This hurts, I'm tired, and I need a break."

As you get older, you generally learn to listen to your body, and are better able to discern between fatigue, which I'll label "good pain," and injury, also known as "bad pain." I've found that the most common cause of injury is performing an exercise incorrectly. In addition to improper form, using too much weight, overtraining, not warming up adequately, and not recognizing one's limitations can all add up to injury.

You can prevent many physical injuries if you just watch for your body's signs. This chapter shows you how to recognize some of your body's warning signals.

Are You Ready to Begin Exercising?

You don't need to see all of those disclaimers on every piece of exercise equipment like, "Consult your physician before using," to know that you should see your doctor and get a physical before starting any exercise program. This is especially true if you're body is deconditioned (see Chapter 8). Common sense tells you it's a good idea to consult a professional.

Maybe you're not quite sure if you're deconditioned. Give yourself a quick test by walking up a flight of stairs. If you're breathing heavily, you're probably not in great shape. If your heavy breathing isn't enough to get you to your doc's office, take a look at your family history. Have any of your relatives had heart disease, strokes, high blood pressure, high cholesterol, diabetes, or a tendency to obesity? If so, you should see your physician for a thorough health exam or your yearly physical. Many medical treatments allow you to exercise safely, and such treatments may decrease the likelihood that you'll significantly disable yourself when you start an exercise program.

Start out slowly

Your body is much like a factory. You need to acquire the proper equipment and take time to train the workers in order to put out quality products. If you look at your body as a moving factory, you can see that to build your muscles, you need to develop your internal machinery. As you gradually build your muscles, they'll produce proteins that enable them to become bigger and stronger — and the more efficient your body factory is, the better it runs.

Of course, just like building up a factory, developing your muscles takes time. In the first four to six weeks of working out, you'll make small gains. Don't give up. The magic is just about to begin. The initial four weeks of working out is the amount of time it takes to develop the machinery to build more muscle. During those first few weeks, take it easy and start off slowly. Your body will not respond well to heavy exercise, especially if you are deconditioned. If you jump in to a program full force, without giving your body a chance to adjust to the stress you're putting on it, you'll probably end up either very sore, injured, or at the very least missing your next couple of workouts. I've even seen people totally give up on a new workout program because they didn't work their way into it.

At this point in their workout frustration, I like to bring up the tortoise and the hare story. Remember the ending? The tortoise won the race because he took his time, was patient and consistent in his pursuit, and kept his goal in mind. So, during the first four to six weeks of your new program, remember the tortoise and concentrate on performing your exercises correctly, improving your flexibility, maintaining a healthy diet, and giving your body a sufficient amount of rest. After this initial period, your muscles are better adapted to take on a heavier, more intense workout. You'll also be more comfortable and familiar with your workout program, which enables you to perform the exercises correctly and safely.

Listen to your pain

Almost everyone has heard the phrase, "No pain, no gain." What most people don't know is the definition of pain. Pain is the body's warning sign that it's in jeopardy of being injured. A more appropriate phase would be, "If it hurts, don't do it." You may be performing an exercise incorrectly, or the exercise may not work well for you. Pain may also indicate that you have an injury you are aggravating by the exercise you are performing. Back in high school I injured my left shoulder. It seemed to have healed, but years later I was doing a bench press (a chest exercise) and felt pain in my shoulder. The assistance my shoulder gave to complete this exercise caused my old injury to act up and created the pain I was feeling. I found another exercise to replace the bench press and I have not incurred any more shoulder pain.

Know How Far to Take It

This may sound like unusual advice, but if you're not reaching the point of failure in your workout, you're not getting the most out of it. What I mean by failure follows: During your muscle conditioning exercises, you should gradually increase the amount of weight you're lifting — enough repetitions that you exhaust or deplete your energy to lift it one more time.

If you've already been working out for several months and you're performing your exercises correctly, your next step is to get the most out of each workout. The best way to stimulate muscle growth and strength is to push your muscles to a new level. This can be accomplished by changing exercises, increasing your weights, increasing the intensity of your workout (by decreasing the time interval between sets, for example), and pushing your muscles to the point of fatigue or failure. Serious athletes constantly use all of these techniques to adapt their muscles to new stresses.

Remember, in order for your muscles to grow, you need to fatigue them. This simply means that with all your effort you can't perform one more repetition of the exercise, even if the guy next to you offered you the winning lottery ticket. So next time you're conditioning your muscles, play a little mind game with yourself and pretend that someone is working out with you (and yes, you can choose any*body* that motivates you). Your partner is offering you a million dollars for each repetition you perform past your goal. If the good-looking imaginary body next to you doesn't motivate you, the million should help you to pull off a few more reps.

Know When to Quit

Even if you're doing everything right, it is possible to overtrain. Overtraining means that you are exercising in excess of your body's capacity to repair itself or adapt to the stresses you present it. It's often difficult to ascertain whether or not you are overtraining. This is when it's really important to listen to your body. If you are overtraining, your body's repair mechanisms are overloaded and you're in prime position for injury. Common but subtle signs of overtraining are as follows:

- ✔ Losing strength

- ✔ Feeling tired in the gym

- ✔ Losing motivation to work out

- ✔ Simply feeling burned out

- ✔ Contracting illnesses such as colds and the flu

- ✔ Experiencing an elevated heart rate when walking at a normal pace

- ✔ Going through uncharacteristic depression

Another way you can determine if you're over-training is to monitor your *resting heart rate* (see Chapter 10 for heart rate charts). If you find an increase in your *resting* heart rate, whether you're continuing your workouts at the same level or at an increased level of intensity, it's time to back off. You may be laughing now, thinking to yourself, "Right, like I have to worry about overtraining when I don't know how I'm going to get off this couch."

Assuming you *do* plan on getting off the couch, use this method to check your progress. Begin by taking your resting heart rate first thing in the morning. As soon as you wake up, roll over, look at the clock, and take your heart rate for one minute (see Chapter 10 for directions). Record your heart rate and keep it for future reference.

In general, the higher your resting heart rate, the less physically fit you are, and the lower your heart rate, the more physically fit you are. (Some athletes have resting heart rates in the 40s.) One way to see if you're working out too much is to check your resting heart rate over a few months. See if it has increased, decreased, or remained the same. If your workouts are effective, your resting heart rate will slowly decrease, or at least remain constant. Your body has many ways of telling you when enough is enough, and if your resting heart rate has increased, you should start listening to your body by decreasing your workout frequency or intensity.

Avoiding Injuries

Overtraining can lead to injuries. If you get injured, you're likely to quit exercising and never work out again. This isn't good. Your body needs to exercise just like it needs to sleep and eat.

The following list of Do's and Don'ts helps you avoid unnecessary injuries.

- ✔ **Do watch** for your body's warning signs and signals.
- ✔ **Do perform the exercise correctly.** (Check the *Tips* and *Caution* sections after each exercise in this book.)
- ✔ **Do warm up and stretch** before and after exercising.
- ✔ **Do start out slowly** and gradually increase your workouts. (Have you heard this enough?)
- ✔ **Do relax,** breathe, and take time to enjoy your life.
- ✔ **Don't jump into an exercise** too quickly.
- ✔ **Don't overdo** an activity.
- ✔ **Do get proper rest** between exercise sessions.
- ✔ **Do use proper body mechanics** when lifting objects or executing sports skills.
- ✔ **Don't exercise when you're ill or overtrained.**
- ✔ **Don't return to your normal exercise program** until your athletic injuries have healed.

Injuries only put you out of commission and into depression. When your body hurts, your mind goes into a state of depression, making it hard to enjoy any aspect of daily life. Anything good takes time, so take your workouts on a step-by-step basis and you'll soon reach your goals.

Part II
My Body Type's Best Workout

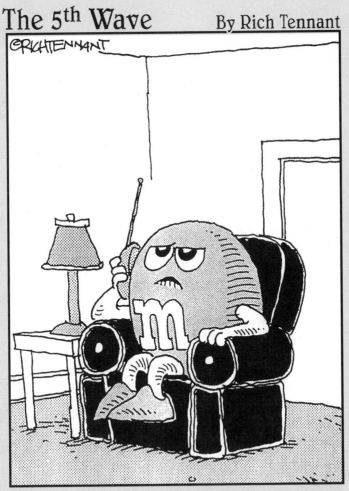

"My body type? I'm an 'M.' But I'd like to get down to an 'N,' maybe an 'H.'"

In this part . . .

This part is where the real fun starts. I give you all the information you need to determine what type of body you have. Each type (mesomorph, ectomorph, or endomorph body shapes) is described in one chapter so that you can review them to find out which one best matches your own. I also provide tests in this part to help you to determine your fitness level and create a workout program specifically designed for your body.

Chapter 5

The Mesomorph Body Type

In This Chapter

▶ Examining the mesomorph body type

▶ Determining your mesomorph type

▶ Discovering the good and bad mesomorph traits

▶ Designing your mesomorph workout

*I*n this chapter I define the most prominent characteristics of the mesomorph body type. You figure out how your body responds to exercise, what sports you're a natural for, and what you're not so great at (and yes, there are a couple of things), plus the best forms of exercise to make you look and feel great.

TAMILEE SAYS

I am a mesomorph and my husband also happens to have this body type. Mesomorphs are usually built to perform athletically, which makes us a perfect match for each other. We both enjoy being physically active and playing sports, and we're pretty equal in our athletic abilities. Well, except in basketball, where I always win!

What Is a Mesomorph?

LINGO

A mesomorph (or meso, for short) can be defined in one word: muscular (see Figure 5-1, or for a female mesomorph, Figure 5-2). If you're a meso, your body type is usually the envy of all gym rats (gym-goers) because you can increase your muscle size quickly and easily. The well-developed, rectangular shapes of mesomorphs are representative of their thick bones and muscles. (Before you get too excited about this perfect form, keep in mind that being a meso may also mean you have poor flexibility.) If you are a characteristic mesomorph, you have a well-defined chest and shoulders that are both larger and broader than your waistline. Your abdomen is taut and your hips are generally the same width as your shoulders. Your buttocks, thighs, and calves are all toned and defined. By the way, if this perfectly describes you, stop reading and give this book to someone who needs it. Chances are, though, that you don't have all the features of a characteristic mesomorph, but rather a blend of features from other body types, too.

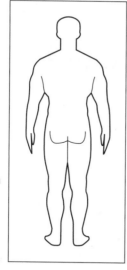

Figure 5-1:
The typical
mesomorph
body type.

As muscularly defined, athletic-looking individuals, mesomorphs are full of energy, are physically capable of a lot of activity, and tend to be aggressive athletically. (Usually no couch potatoes in this group.) Although mesomorphs generally store fat evenly all over their bodies, they can become overweight if they are sedentary and consume a high-fat and/or high-calorie diet. Cardiovascular disease can be a primary threat to an overweight meso, so if you fit into that category, your best method of prevention is to maintain a healthy diet and a balanced exercise regime. Remember that your heart is a muscle too, and the best way to keep it fit is to perform cardiovascular activities. (See Chapter 9 for cardiovascular workouts.)

Craving physical activity and constantly seeking action, the mesomorph makes a great athlete. As a meso, you excel in sports that require great strength, short bursts of energy, and lots of power. Mesos are always popular in gym class and at the playground, because people want mesos on their teams. If you're scouting for body types at your local gym (and who isn't?), you will most likely find your fellow mesos lifting weights and avoiding the cardio equipment like step machines or treadmills.

When you think "mesomorph," think of Sylvester Stallone and Demi Moore.

Sports and activities

If you are a mesomorph, you may enjoy participating in these sports. After all, your body type is naturally suited for these activities. (If you aren't a meso, you can find a list of sports that you may prefer in Chapters 6 and 7, which describe other body types.) You may have noticed similarities in the physical requirements for the sports listed. Muscle mass is at the top of the list of requirements. The majority of these activities also demand strong muscles, short bursts of energy, and powerful full body movements.

If you've ever tried ballet, runway fashion modeling, or long-distance running, you probably already figured out that as a mesomorph, a few things in life may not come easily to you. These activities are best suited for someone with an ectomorph body type (see Chapter 6 for more on ectomorphs). By no means do we mean that you can't be anything you want to be. It's just that you may find out you have to work a little harder to participate in certain activities. Never give up hope — just about any athletic goal is possible if you want it and are willing to work for it.

- Baseball
- Bicycling
- Boxing
- Diving
- Football (especially linemen and backs)
- Golf
- Gymnastics
- Judo
- Lacrosse
- Rugby
- Shot and discus
- Speed skating
- Sprinting (track and field)
- Weight lifting
- Wrestling

A Test to Determine What Type of Meso You Are

Three levels of the mesomorph body type are shown (see Figure 5-2). Both men and women mesomorphs have well-defined muscle, but the male mesomorph is proportionately larger in both muscle and bone mass. Try to match your meso body up with one of the figures. Figure 5-2 also shows the ectomorph and endomorph body types to help you see the differences.

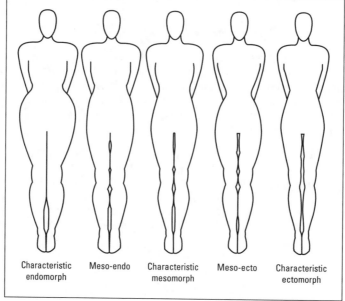

| Characteristic endomorph | Meso-endo | Characteristic mesomorph | Meso-ecto | Characteristic ectomorph |

Figure 5-2: The characteristic ecto and endo body types with the mesomorph body types.

The meso-ecto body

Moving toward the ectomorph body type on the scale is the meso-ecto body type (refer to Figure 5-2). As a meso-ecto, you generally have a smaller bone frame, but carry a meso's muscle size and build. You have a tendency to be lean like your ectomorph neighbors, yet your natural abilities for strength are greater than that of the endurance-built ectomorph. (See Chapter 6 for more details on ectomorphs.)

The characteristic mesomorph body

Sitting in the middle of the scale is the characteristic mesomorph (shown in Figure 5-2). You find these bodies amongst the patrons of California's popular Muscle Beach — with thick muscle mass and bones, characteristic mesomorphs are sure to stand out in a crowd. Structurally, if you're a characteristic meso, your chest and hips tend to be wide, and you have an allover rectangular frame. Typically, more men than women have this large frame mesomorph body type.

The meso-endo body

Just to the left of the characteristic meso on the scale in Figure 5-2 you find the meso-endo body type. As a meso-endo, you have the ability to retain a great deal of muscle mass but may have a tendency to carry a little extra body fat, which is a characteristic trait of the endomorph body type (see Chapter 7 for more information on endomorphs). Typically the extra body fat is evenly distributed throughout the meso-endo body, but by increasing cardiovascular exercise you can maintain a healthy body weight.

Facts: The Good, the Bad, but Never the Ugly

You have to take the good with the bad, so be optimistic and make your body the best it can be. Remember, as a mesomorph, you have the muscle on your side. So how can you lose?

The good mesomorph traits

You have an ability to put on muscle easily, which is beneficial to anyone trying to maintain a healthy body weight. By increasing your muscle mass, you increase your body's metabolism. This is positive because when your metabolism is higher you burn more calories while sitting on the couch than a person, with a similar body type, who has less muscle mass.

Increasing your metabolism is an incentive in itself, but remember that strong muscles also help support your skeletal frame. Maintaining strong muscles is especially important as you age. Your bones naturally decrease in density as you get older. Strong, flexible muscles can help to support the body's frame and prevent injury.

Muscle makes the body look shapely. Tone, firm arms, abdominals (we call them abs for short), buttocks, and legs create a curvy hourglass figure. There's no need for shoulder pads on your mesomorph body.

It has finally become a trend for women to show off the muscles they have. Women who shape and tone their bodies can be found in the limelight in music videos and women's sports teams. Women like Janet Jackson and Madonna make it a point to show their strong arms and abs. Gabrielle Reese, who is a balanced meso, shows the world her talents as a star volleyball player and at the same time graces the covers of several magazines, exhibiting the beauty of muscle. Contrary to popular belief, women who weight train do not look like men. Even the female mesomorph, who builds muscle naturally and easily, never becomes big and bulky like her male counterpart without the use of illegal drugs, such as steroids, to enhance the body.

The bad mesomorph traits

Unfortunately, some mesomorphs do have a tendency to carry fat almost as easily as they do muscle. If this trend is a problem for you, you can quickly remedy it by increasing your cardiovascular workouts to combat the fat. Fortunately, because mesomorphs have more metabolically active muscle tissue, losing weight with aerobic exercise (which burns calories) is easier to do than for people with other body types.

Due to their thick bones and muscles, mesomorphs may look heavier than they actually are. Purchasing clothing that fits can also be a difficult task for you. Men may have to wear custom-made suits due to their large chests and arm widths. Women who have large thigh and calf muscles may find it difficult to find jeans that fit comfortably. Those of you who face this dilemma, please feel free to curse Calvin Klein and his jeans.

Last, you must always work on maintaining flexibility. Thick muscles may tend to be tight muscles, so keep them limber. (See Chapter 3 for a stretch routine.)

Dress to enhance your mesomorph figure

If your figure has an hourglass shape or your hips and shoulders are the same width and your waist is narrow, you can enhance your figure by:

✔ Wearing vertical stripes, which help create a longer, leaner silhouette.

✔ Wearing clothes that lie loosely on your hips and chest. Avoid tight pants or jeans.

✔ Avoiding clothes that place horizontal lines across your chest or rear end.

Mesomorph Workouts

In this section I show you some sample workout schedules for each of the mesomorph body types. I also help you design the program that works best for you.

A general recommendation for all mesomorphs is to set a goal to work out 3 to 4 times per week. When you are designing your workout program, do your best to incorporate cardiovascular activity (see Chapter 9), muscle toning exercises (see Chapters 10 through 15), and stretching (see Chapter 3).

Your workouts can be broken down into $1/2$ hour increments each day, or you may choose to combine your cardio and toning exercises within the same day. For example, if you plan to work out 3 days during the week you may want to do both your cardio and toning workouts each of the 3 days. If you can fit in more days for your workouts, try alternating your activities from day to day. While doing your cardiovascular routines, try to reach 55 to 90 percent of your maximum heart rate (see Chapter 9 for heart rate charts). You can be the judge of your muscle conditioning workouts. If you put on muscle quickly and easily, you may not need to do a conditioning workout more than 1 to 2 days a week. Overall, listen to your body. It will tell you when enough is enough. Muscle soreness the next day or two is normal, but if you feel pain or become injured, take a break. That's your body telling you that you need to ease off from your workouts. *Note:* If you are overtraining, your body may give you warning signs like a decrease in your ability to perform. You may also get a cold, the flu, or cold sores on your lips, which can mean that your immune system is depressed from inadequate recovery time in between your workouts.

Muscles need time to repair and rebuild. Avoid strength training the same muscle group 2 days in a row. Muscle fibers break down during a workout, and as they mend themselves naturally they increase in size. A good recommendation is to give each muscle group a 48-hour rest between workouts. (Not 48 days!) For example, if you exercised your biceps on Monday, you should wait until at least Wednesday before you exercise them again.

Why do my muscles get sore after my workout?

Your muscles are made up of millions of small fibers called myofibrils. Some of these fibers break under the tension of exercise and release chemicals that make your muscles sore. These same chemicals stimulate the body to repair the myofibrils and add a few more. This process increases your muscle size and better prepares your muscles to do the same activity again.

Meso-ecto general workout routine

Muscle strength and conditioning = 50 percent of your total workout time

Cardiovascular activity   = 50 percent of your total workout time

Example: Your schedule allows you to work out 3 days a week. You need to balance your routine so that you do equal amounts of cardio and muscle toning exercises. Each of the three days, you allot 2 hours to work out, for a total workout time of 6 hours each week. As long as you are exercising aerobically for 3 of those hours and toning your muscles for the other 3 hours, you can mix and match your programs any way you choose.

For example, you can do 1 hour of cardio and 1 hour of muscle toning on Mondays, 2 hours of cardio on Thursdays, and 2 hours of muscle toning on Saturdays. Your cardio exercises can consist of a step machine workout, a bike ride, or a walk or jog. All of your cardio workouts should be programmed for endurance rather than toning. This is because your body naturally puts on muscle easily, so when you are performing cardiovascular exercises, you want to focus on exercising your heart. The rest of your muscles develop easily with the muscle conditioning exercises. (See Chapters 9 through 15 for specific muscle-conditioning and cardiovascular exercises.)

Characteristic mesomorph general workout routine

Muscle strength and conditioning = 40 percent of your total workout time

Cardiovascular activity   = 60 percent of your total workout time

Example: To maintain a healthy body fat percentage, working out aerobically 4 to 5 times per week is best. Your body builds muscle easily so your weight-training program requires a little less time than your cardio program.

For example, your normal routine may be to get a $1^1/_2$ hour workout 5 days a week. That makes your total workout time $7^1/_2$ hours each week. 60 percent of those hours (approximately 4 hours), you cross train for your cardiovascular workouts, so you take spinning classes (see Chapter 9 for more on this activity), run, or in-line skate. The other 40 percent of the workout time ($3^1/_2$ hours), you do heavy weight lifting exercises. (See Chapters 9 through 15 for muscle-conditioning and cardiovascular exercises.)

Meso-endo general workout routine

Muscle strength and conditioning = 40 percent of your total workout time

Cardiovascular activity = 60 percent of your total workout time

Example: Your body may have a tendency to carry a little extra body fat so it would be wise to focus a bit more of your workout time doing cardiovascular exercises. Fortunately, having mesomorph qualities you can gain muscle easily so you can spend less time conditioning your muscles. A good goal to set for yourself would be to work out 4 to 5 times per week doing some type of cardiovascular endurance training activity and then incorporate your muscle conditioning exercises 1 to 2 days during the week.

For example, you may plan your workouts for Monday through Friday. On each of those days you spend an hour doing your cardio workout, such as jogging or biking. You also add an extra hour to two of those days to work on conditioning your muscles. (See Chapters 9 through 15 for muscle-conditioning and cardiovascular exercises.)

Most people enjoy doing things they are naturally good at. As a mesomorph, you're probably no exception. You may gravitate toward weight lifting over cardiovascular exercise due to your ease in building muscle. *Remember:* You need a balanced workout routine that combines the three necessary components of fitness:

- ✔ Muscle conditioning
- ✔ Cardiovascular activity
- ✔ Flexibility (See Chapter 3 for more on this topic.)

Chapter 6

Life as an Ectomorph

In This Chapter

▶ Examining the ectomorph body type

▶ Determining which type of ectomorph you are

▶ Discovering the good and bad ectomorph traits

▶ Designing your ectomorph workout

*I*n this chapter I define the traits of the ectomorph body type. You also figure out which sports and activities are best suited for you, as well as how to keep your physique trim, toned, and healthy.

TAMILEE SAYS

Lori Seeger (my associate and writer of this book) has traveled with me for several years, assisting me at my lectures and workshops. I wish I had a dollar for every person who approaches us and asks, "Are you two sisters?" We do admit that we have similar taste in clothing and hair color, but if you really look at us, you can see we have very different body types. Lori leads the life of an ectomorph, while I, on the other hand, am a purebred mesomorph (defined in Chapter 5). Lori has long legs and enjoys running, but has a tough time increasing her muscle mass. I have short legs and despise running, but have won women's weight-lifting competitions. It has been rumored that if you spend a lot of time with someone you begin to speak and dress similarly, but I can assure you that my legs have not gotten any longer in the past six years, and I'm sure I'll never choose running as my favorite exercise.

What Is an Ectomorph?

LINGO

A one-word description for the ectomorph body type (or *ecto,* for short) is *slim* (see Figure 6-1 for an example of a male ectomorph, and Figure 6-2 for a female ectomorph). If you're an ecto, mesomorphs and endomorphs (see Chapters 5 and 7) usually don't want to stand next to you. It's not that ectomorphs aren't personable, it's just that you're probably a tall, slender individual who has trouble gaining weight (oh darn!). As you may have guessed, the perfect example of an ecto is a fashion model.

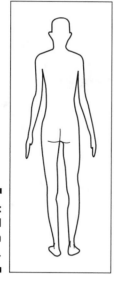

Figure 6-1:
The typical
ectomorph
body type.

An ectomorph is relatively linear in shape with a delicate build, narrow hips and pelvis, and long arms and legs. As an ecto, your muscle and bone outlines are usually visible (especially if you are an extremely thin ecto), and you normally have less fat and muscle mass than people with other body types. Remember, though, that you probably don't have all of the features of a characteristic endomorph, but a blend of features from more than one body type.

Although willowy ectomorphs cover the majority of fashion magazines, nobody's perfect, and ectos do have health concerns. Your primary concern as an ectomorph is your frail stature consisting of small bones and joints that have a tendency to be injured easily during sporting activities.

So what I'm trying to tell you is that you probably won't be the star of your football team or the next champion gladiator. Don't worry — your body type is naturally suited to perform wonderfully in endurance activities. Just remember: balancing your activities is the key. Like mesomorphs (see Chapter 15 for a description of this body type), ectos have a tendency to stick with what they do best, and ectos excel at cardiovascular training. You find balance in your workouts when you do both aerobic and muscle training.

When you think "ectomorph," think of Tom Hanks and Courtney Cox.

Sports and activities

The following list is a series of sports and activities you may enjoy participating in if you're an ectomorph. You may notice that each activity requires cardiovascular strength, agility, speed, and precision movements. If you're an ectomorph, try one of these activities — you may find out that you're pretty good at them. Check out Chapters 5 and 7 to see sports you may enjoy if you are a mesomorph or endomorph.

- ✔ Ballet
- ✔ Basketball
- ✔ Cycling
- ✔ Dance
- ✔ Diving
- ✔ Marathon or long distance running

- ✔ Racquetball
- ✔ Rock climbing
- ✔ Swimming
- ✔ Track and field (hurdles, high and long jumps)
- ✔ Volleyball

A Test to Determine What Type of Ecto You Are

Ectomorphs, although generally possessing longer, thinner muscles, can be very strong. Muscle tissue on ectos is very defined but usually never thick and bulky like the mesomorph body type (see Chapter 5 for more on mesos). Try to match your ecto body with one of the figures in Figure 6-2, which shows the characteristic endomorph and mesomorph types next to levels of the ectomorph body type.

The characteristic ectomorph body

Do you remember Popeye's girlfriend, Olive Oyl? She's the ecto of all ectos, and probably can't put on a pound of weight even if she ate Popeye's spinach. This ectomorph body type is shown in Figure 6-2. Generally, as a characteristic ecto, you have a great deal of difficulty putting on muscle or weight in general. You may tend to look thin and bony and have a frail skeletal structure.

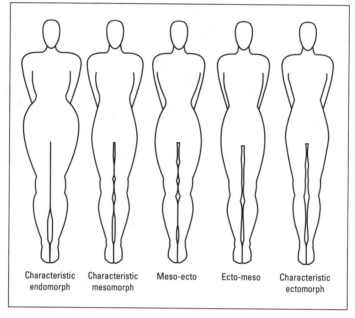

Figure 6-2:
The
characteristic
endo and
meso next
to the
ectomorph
body types.

Characteristic endomorph | Characteristic mesomorph | Meso-ecto | Ecto-meso | Characteristic ectomorph

The ecto-meso, a fashion designer's dream model

The ecto-meso (refer to Figure 6-2) has all the qualities of a balanced ecto plus a slight blending of mesomorph traits (see Chapter 5).

Although as an ecto-meso you have an ability to add some muscle mass with strength-training exercises, your body most likely has long, lean muscles. Long-distance runners are a good example of this body type. You also see some fashion models, such as Cindy Crawford, who are able to develop and tone their muscles plus have all the qualities of the lean ecto body.

The meso-ecto body type

Yes it's true: Some people are born rich, some with exceptional intelligence, and some with naturally beautiful bodies. The meso-ecto, positioned between the mesomorph body type and the ecto-meso on the scale in Figure 6-2, has what many people want . . . a body that easily develops muscle tone and generally has little difficulty decreasing excess body fat. The combination of mesomorph (see Chapter 5) and ectomorph traits tend to make this body type one of the most desired physiques.

The Best of Times, the Worst of Times as an Ectomorph

Every body type has its good and bad traits. Take the features you've been given and make your body the best it can be. After all, you're starting off with some pretty fine traits. So take a moment to admire some of those fine physical qualities, and use them to motivate you to work on the parts you're not so enthused about. You may be surprised at what a little hard work can do to help you achieve your goals.

The good ectomorph traits

The naturally thin ectomorph body has relatively little body fat. For overall health, this is one of the finest qualities of being an ecto. As an ecto, one of the reasons that you have a naturally low amount of body fat is because your metabolism tends to be faster than that of a mesomorph or endomorph (see Chapters 5 and 7 for information on the metabolism of these body types) — which enables you to burn more calories even at rest. In addition, your inherent capacity for aerobic endurance is the sign of a strong cardiovascular system and helps you, as an ectomorph, maintain your lean body. If that isn't enough, your muscles and joints are also naturally flexible, which aids in injury prevention as you age.

So, you think that as an ecto you can eat whatever you want (like triple fudge chocolate cake) and never gain any weight? Sorry to disappoint you, but this is a myth. Ectos may appear to be thin on the exterior, but if you don't work out and take care of your body, you'll be fat on the inside. The down side is that if you don't exercise and you consume a high-fat diet, you are placing yourself in risk of causing an insulin resistance in your body, which may lead to increased dangers: cholesterol, HDL and LDL, hypertension, and obesity. Keep in mind that being *thin* doesn't always mean that you're healthy. If you're taking care of your interior health, you'll be rewarded with a beautiful exterior body.

The bad ectomorph traits

To some people, having trouble *gaining* weight may seem like winning the lottery, but to many ectomorphs this problem is a constant struggle. You know what I'm talking about if you've ever heard people say they eat whatever they want and never gain weight. This may sound like it's not a problem at all, but in fact, the inability to gain weight may indicate a serious health problem such as thyroid dysfunction or diabetes.

> ## Dress to enhance your ectomorph figure
>
> If you feel you can fit your figure in a rectangle and fill it up equally, you probably have shoulders, a waist, and hips that are approximately the same width. In order to create a more shapely silhouette, you could:
>
> ✔ Wear a belt or a top or bottom that gathers at the waist.
>
> ✔ Wear open jackets or tops.

For men, having an ecto body can be synonymous with being wimpy or being the guy who gets sand kicked in his face, which is why weight training is beneficial to gain muscle size and strength.

The struggle doesn't stop there, though, because general muscle growth takes longer, too. As an ectomorph, if you don't add muscle-toning exercises to your workout regimen, you may have a higher fat to muscle ratio.

Ectomorph Workouts

This section is geared to give you a sample workout schedule if you are a characteristic ecto, an ecto-meso, or a meso-ecto. Then I help you design a program that works best for you.

A general goal for all ectomorphs is to work out 3 to 4 times a week. Your workouts should consist of cardiovascular activity (see Chapter 9 for cardio exercises), muscle-toning exercises (see Chapters 10 through 15 for suggestions), and stretching (see Chapter 3 for stretch routines). Combining these three components of fitness is not only essential for a balanced workout, but also helpful in adding variety to your activities.

You can mix, match, and break up your workouts however you choose. For instance, if you work out 2 or 3 days a week, you may want to combine your cardio and muscle-toning workouts each day. If you have four or more days to work your body, you may choose to alternate activities, like cardio on 2 days and muscle toning the other 2 days. During your cardiovascular routines, try to reach 55 to 90 percent of your maximum heart rate (see Chapter 8 to learn how to calculate your personal maximum heart rate).

Use them or lose them

Wanting to look like the model on the cover of *Cosmo* or *Men's Health* is the cosmetic side of why you may want to develop and define your muscles. The practical side is simple: If you don't use them, you'll lose them. Your muscles won't vanish into thin air, but you can experience *atrophy,* a condition where your muscles decrease in size and tone due to lack of use. Of course, if you give your muscles what they're asking for (strength and endurance training, in case you didn't know), you may experience hypertrophy. *Hypertrophy* is an increase in muscle mass and strength.

Ectomorphs in particular are more likely to achieve muscle hypertrophy from exercising with heavier weights and less repetitions while conditioning their muscles.

When strength-training your muscles, however, you must remember to give them time to rest and repair themselves. You'll achieve your best results by skipping a day in between your weight lifting workouts. If you have time you can certainly work out every day, but don't strength train *each* muscle daily. Every muscle needs time to rest.

Muscles need time to rebuild. Muscle fibers break down during a workout, and as they mend themselves naturally, they increase in size. A good recommendation is to give each muscle group a 48-hour rest between workouts.

The meso-ecto general workout routine

Muscle strength and conditioning = 50 percent of your total workout time

Cardiovascular activity = 50 percent of your total workout time

Example: You can balance your workout by performing equal amounts of muscle conditioning and cardiovascular exercises. If you choose to work out 4 days a week with a total exercise time of 6 hours, you could spend 3 hours doing cardiovascular exercises like running and cycling (see Chapter 9 for more cardio exercises) and 3 hours lifting weights in the gym (see Chapters 10 through 15 for muscle conditioning exercises).

The ecto-meso general workout routine

Muscle strength and conditioning = 60 percent of your total workout time

Cardiovascular activity = 40 percent of your total workout time

Example: You need to spend more time increasing your muscle mass. Suppose that you have only 3 days a week to exercise for a total workout time of 3 hours. You try to spend up to 2 of those hours building your muscles (see Chapters 10 through 15 for suggestions), and an hour to an hour and a half doing cardio activity like running on a treadmill or in-line skating. (See Chapter 9 for cardio workouts.)

The characteristic ectomorph general workout routine

Muscle strength and conditioning = 60 percent of your total workout time

Cardiovascular activity = 40 percent of your total workout time

Example: Your goal is definitely to increase your muscle mass. Try to spend the larger percentage of your exercise time doing muscle-conditioning exercises (see Chapters 10 through 15 for suggestions), but don't forget to condition your heart, too, with cardio activity like walking, in-line skating, or biking. (See Chapter 9 for information on cardio workouts.) For example, if you only have time to work out 2 or 3 days a week, try to do some sort of muscle-conditioning exercise each day and add your cardio workout on top of that.

If you find yourself doing mostly cardio activity instead of training your muscles, reassess your workout plan. As an ecto, you are naturally good at endurance activities and will find yourself gravitating towards them.

Chapter 7

The Endomorph Body Type

*R*emember the days when Marilyn Monroe had the figure that most women (and men) craved? This memory brings to mind a figure that represents an endomorph body type. This curvaceous body type is represented in the statues of great sculptors, the paintings of famous artists, and in Hollywood by many actresses.

This chapter is designed to help you identify the traits of the endomorph body type. I let you in on which activities you perform well and give you tips for making your body the best it can be.

What is an Endomorph?

A one-word description of the endomorph body type (or endo, for short) is curvy (see Figure 7-1). The soft, flowing curves of an endo are similar to that of an hourglass in more ways than one. And wouldn't you know it; the sands of an hourglass tend to settle in its bottom half just like the fat in the body. Comparatively, if you're an endomorph, your body fat may have a tendency to settle into the lower regions of your body, predominantly the lower abdomen, hips, and thighs, rather than being distributed evenly throughout your body. Keep in mind, though, that most endomorphs don't have all the features of characteristic endomorph, but a blend of features from other body types as well.

Most people like to read the not-so-good stuff before the good stuff, so first I give the "bad" news to you straight, and then I tell you the good parts. I also tell you how to make the not-so-good part better.

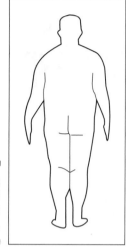

Figure 7-1:
The typical
endomorph
body type.

An endomorph body typically has the capacity for high fat storage, and unfortunately puts fat on pretty easily. Although all body types are susceptible to excessive weight gain, as an endomorph, you are more inclined to become obese. The majority of your body weight is either centered in the middle of your body or in your hip and buttocks regions. You know what I'm referring to if you ever have the feeling that every time you gain weight it jumps right to your butt. A fruit shape metaphor frequently used to describe an endomorph body type is a pear. A pear resembles a body that has more weight in the lower region, like the hips and thighs, than the upper portion of the body. Structurally, as an endo you have small to medium bones, limbs that are shorter in relation to your trunk, and musculature that is not well defined.

Now for the good news. From top to bottom, your soft swelling curves create full, rounded shoulders, limbs, and a full trunk. Voluptuous and sensual are the descriptions given to many endomorph females whose soft body contours and deep curves create an allure like that of Marilyn Monroe. See? I told you there is good stuff.

A male endomorph (known as an android) tends to have a different fat distribution pattern from a female endomorph (known as a gynoid). Female endos usually collect fat in their butts, legs, and hips, while most males collect fat in their abdomen (the "spare tire" or "love handle" look). Many research studies have shown that abdominal fat deposition is much more dangerous than fat in the leg and butt area. This is primarily due to the danger of heart disease and an increased risk of diabetes, stroke, some cancers, and high blood pressure.

Sports and activities

Endomorphs are best suited for heavy-contact sports. The following list shows some sports and activities you may enjoy. (See Chapters 5 and 6 for sports you may excel in if you're a mesomorph or ectomorph.) Strength, a lower center of gravity, and an ability to exert power from the lower portion of the body are all advantageous when performing these activities. Water activities are also good for this body type because endomorph bodies have a tendency to float better and do not drag or become excessively weighted in the water.

- Cricket
- Football (defensive line)
- Golf
- Judo
- Lacrosse
- Racquetball
- Rugby
- Softball
- Squash
- Recreational swimming
- Tennis
- Track and field (shot and discus)
- Water polo
- Weight lifting (heavy)
- Wrestling (heavy weight)

The key to taking the bad with the good and finding happiness with your body type is by balancing all aspects of your life. Your first concern is your health, and your major health concern as an endo is maintaining a healthy body weight. Excessive amounts of body fat can place you in jeopardy of cardiovascular disease. Remember that the risk of such disease is increased if the majority of the fat is carried in the center of your body surrounding your heart. This danger can easily be avoided by maintaining a healthy diet and exercising. (See Chapter 8 to find out how to design your own exercise program.) The joints of your lower body may be another health concern. Because these joints are already highly susceptible to injury, high-impact sports or activities may be damaging to them, especially if you carry excess body weight.

When you think "endomorph," think of Robin Williams and Oprah Winfrey.

If you're looking for more information on the endomorph body type, check out a book written by Dr. Glenn Gaesser titled *Big Fat Lies: The Truth about your Weight and Health* (Ballantine Books, 1998).

A Test to Determine What Type of Endo You Are

Figure 7-2 shows three levels of the endomorph body type. Each level demonstrates the characteristics of a typical endo, but is separated by the degree to which the body stores fat. Try to match your endo body with one of the samples. Figure 7-2 also shows the mesomorph and ectomorph body types so that you can compare the endomorph to them.

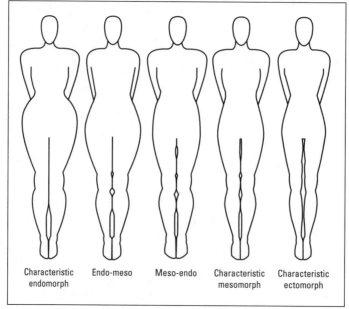

Figure 7-2: The characteristic meso and ecto body types next to the endomorph types.

| Characteristic endomorph | Endo-meso | Meso-endo | Characteristic mesomorph | Characteristic ectomorph |

The powerfully curvy meso-endo body

The meso-endo body type (refer to Figure 7-2) has the ability to increase muscle mass quite easily due to its mesomorph characteristic (see Chapter 5 for more information on mesomorphs), but it also may have difficulty losing excess body fat because it carries traits of the endomorph. Unlike the characteristic endomorph, whose excess weight is generally found from the hips to the lower legs, the meso-endo usually gains weight evenly throughout the body. Although the overall silhouette of a meso-endo is evenly proportioned with muscle and fat, the muscle will not appear lean and defined unless this person focuses on maintaining a low body fat percentage with cardiovascular exercise.

The voluptuous endo-meso body

The endo-meso body type (shown in Figure 7-2) has full, smooth curves and an hourglass waistline. The characteristics distinguishing endo-mesos from balanced endos are broader shoulders, body curves that are more pronounced and firm with muscle mass, and a more prominent chest. If you look at paintings from the Renaissance period, you find this body type is the most popular female figure.

The characteristic endomorph body

Reaching the left of the scale in Figure 7-2, characteristic endos tend to maintain a higher body fat percentage then all other body types. These individuals may be physically strong (like the defensive linemen on a football team), but they do have a higher fat to muscle ratio and must place emphasis on cardiovascular exercise to maintain or reach a healthy body weight.

It's Just How You Look at It

Because no such thing as a perfect body exists, you may as well appreciate what you've been given and work on your potential to have a healthy body. May I remind you that not many things are achieved without a little effort? If your goal is to have a balanced body, you must care for your inner health. Contrary to many societal beliefs, a healthy heart and lungs are more important than a skinny or sculpted exterior. By focusing on and taking care of your internal health, your body in turn rewards you with a beautiful exterior in addition to health and happiness.

The good endomorph traits

Endomorphs are physically strong and can generally gain muscle easily. As an endo, you have the ability to put on a great deal of muscle mass through weight training because your body is accustomed to supporting large amounts of fat. As a result, you have greater potential to carry a larger percentage of muscle mass than mesomorphs and ectomorphs (see Chapters 5 and 6 for more on these body types). A perfect example of a toned, healthy endo is Oprah Winfrey. She prioritizes her internal health by maintaining a healthy diet and exercise program. Her external beauty is the reward she receives from caring for her body.

True or False? Endomorphs are doomed to early deaths from cardiovascular disease and cancer. The answer to this question can be either true or false depending on whether the endomorph takes care of his or her body by exercising and eating right. The real truth is that if a person with an endomorph body type participates in aerobic and strength-training exercise and eats sensibly, he won't have significant risk factors for health problems such as high blood pressure, high cholesterol, and diabetes. Although certain genes create a potential for health problems, these problems are not inevitable if you follow a healthy lifestyle. If this is the case, the risk of heart disease and cancer for an endomorph is no greater than that of a person with another body type.

The bad endomorph traits

As an endomorph, you may see your body as the enemy because you spend your life fighting the battle of the bulge. It can be a constant struggle to watch your diet and dedicate yourself to exercising just to maintain a healthy weight. Although this is generally more indicative of the characteristic endo body, all levels of endomorphs fight to keep the weight from creeping up on them. By taking a different perspective on your body's natural traits, you can find some endos who use their bodies to help establish their careers. For example, Michael Dean Perry gained his fame as one of the best defensive lineman in American football. His body (the frame of a characteristic endo) along with his great physical abilities gained him his nickname: *The Fridge.* He not only resembles a fridge — he's just as immovable.

Dress to enhance your endomorph figure

If your body is shaped like a pear (smaller on the top and bigger on the bottom), you can balance your upper body with your lower half by:

✔ Wearing tops that broaden your shoulders (like those containing shoulder pads).

✔ Wearing long jackets to cover your hip area.

✔ Wearing straight skirts, and avoiding those that are gathered at the waist.

✔ Wearing darker colors or solids and avoiding stripes or prints on your bottom half. (Don't draw more attention to an area you don't want people to stare at.)

If your body is wider in your middle region, you can create a more even balance by:

✔ Wearing tops that come down past your waistline. (Don't wear crop tops.)

✔ Wearing loose fitting clothes and wide flowing skirts.

The struggle to lose weight is the biggest frustration for a majority of endomorphs. Body metabolism tends to be slower for endos than for people with other body types, which makes the process of losing weight more challenging.

Endomorph Workouts

This section shows you sample workout schedules for all levels of the endomorph body type. From there I help you design a program that works best for you.

A general goal for people with all body types is to work out 3 to 4 times per week, but as an endo, you're the exception. Your body type needs a bit more time and attention so you should set your goal to 4 or more workouts a week. Breaking up your workouts is fine. The most important thing to remember is to stay active. Cardiovascular activity (see Chapter 9), muscle-toning exercises (see Chapters 10 through 15), and stretching (see Chapter 4) should all be a part of your workout regimen.

Breaking up your workouts can give you more flexibility in your schedule and can make the whole process more fun. Some days you may choose to just take a long walk (or do some other form of aerobic activity) and do your muscle toning on the next day, or you may choose to lump them together in the same day. Cardiovascular endurance training is important in helping you to maintain a healthy body fat percentage, so get in as much cardiovascular exercise as you can and try to reach 65 to 90 percent of your maximum heart rate (see Chapter 9 for heart rate charts and exercise ideas).

Your best choices for exercise are non-weight bearing and low-impact activities. That means no jogging with your kids on your shoulders. Workouts that are low impact help prevent placing excessive strain on your joints. Cardiovascular workouts that are of long duration with a lower intensity are the key, such as walking 30 minutes or more several times a week. These workouts help you burn excess fat and calories. Swimming, biking, or water aerobics can be fun additions to your workout schedule.

Meso-endo general workout routine

Muscle strength and conditioning = 40% of your total workout time

Cardiovascular activity = 60% of your total workout time

What your muscles can do for you

What's the one muscle in your body that you can't do without? It's your heart — the cardiac muscle. In addition to this head honcho muscle, which keeps the blood pumping and flowing throughout your entire body, you have other muscles that help move your body. These muscle types are called *skeletal* and *smooth*.

✔ Skeletal muscles are the ones you can see when you look at yourself (some locations more than others) and are located throughout your body, in your arms, legs, buns, back, and abdominal area. For some people, these muscles may appear firm or pumped up; to others, they may look as though they are swaying in the breeze. These skeletal muscles allow us to perform locomotive skills like running, jumping, skipping, or just lifting our arms up over our heads. These are the muscles I concentrate on in this book.

✔ Smooth muscles give movement to the organs of your digestive, urinary, and reproductive systems as well as the walls of your blood vessels. These are the muscles I didn't create exercises for. You're on your own here.

Example: You don't have much trouble gaining muscle due to your mesomorph traits, so you can limit your muscle conditioning to 40 percent of your workout time or, for example, an hour 3 to 4 days a week. You could do your cardio workouts 6 days a week or more for at least 30 minutes at a time. This type of routine will help you maintain your muscle and keep your body fat low by staying consistent with your cardio exercise.

(See Chapters 10 through 15 for muscle conditioning and cardiovascular exercises.)

Endo-meso general workout routine

Muscle strength and conditioning = 40% of your total workout time

Cardiovascular activity = 60% of your total workout time

Example: Your body type has a bit more muscle than the characteristic endomorph. You still need to fight the excess fat, so you should concentrate 60 percent of your workout time on cardiovascular exercises such as biking, light jogging, and swimming. Your cardio workouts can be done, for example, 6 days a week for 45 minutes or more at a time. You also increase your muscle mass with conditioning exercises, which you could do 3 to 4 days a week.

(See Chapters 10 through 15 for muscle conditioning and cardiovascular exercises.)

Characteristic endomorph general workout routine

Muscle strength and conditioning = 30% of your total workout time

Cardiovascular activity = 70% of your total workout time

Example: You tend to carry most of your body weight in your abdominal area and lower body region. The extra weight you carry makes it difficult to do any type of high impact cardiovascular activity and also places your lower body joints in jeopardy of being injured. In order to lose your excess body fat, your workouts should consist mostly of low impact cardiovascular activities such as walking and swimming. Another important factor in these workouts is the duration. (The key to weight loss for this body type is long duration and low-intensity exercise.) Your cardio exercises, like walking, should have a duration of 45 minutes to an hour and a half. Because cardio is 70 percent of your workout, it would be best to do some type of cardiovascular exercise 7 days a week. In addition, you could add muscle-conditioning exercises to your workout program 3 days a week.

(See Chapters 10 through 15 for muscle-conditioning and cardiovascular exercises.)

 The secret to balancing the endomorph body is to focus on developing muscle proportionately. If you gain weight in your lower half, but your arms and upper body are thin, you should concentrate on upper-body muscle toning. Cardio endurance and building muscle are your two key factors in developing a well-balanced physique inside and out.

And in case you aren't tired of me reminding you, the following list shows you the three necessary components to every workout program.

- ✔ Muscle conditioning
- ✔ Cardiovascular activity
- ✔ Flexibility (see Chapter 3)

Chapter 8

Your Personalized Workout Program

In This Chapter

▶ Evaluating your fitness level

▶ Charting it all

▶ Determining your exercise goals

▶ Choosing your exercises and developing your program

*N*ow is your chance to be creative. I set up some steps to help you develop your own workout schedule based on the exercises from Chapters 9 through 18.

Creating your own workout is the easy part. It's as simple as determining the body type that you have, choosing your favorite exercises and activities, and filling in the blanks on your personal charts. A self-evaluation is a great way to find out what your strengths and weaknesses are. Many people I've spoken to never want to know their weakness. I see them avoiding these telltale signs by skipping their annual checkup from their doctor — and not admitting that their clothing size has increased to a number surpassing the minimum speed limit in their local town. If you've been pretending that your health doesn't matter, now is the time to look at your current level of fitness and make a choice to be honest with yourself and improve your health.

Take a Look at Yourself

I'm sure most of you aren't psyched about standing naked in front of a mirror, measuring what you see, and then putting it into a chart, but I'm not asking you to hang this chart on your refrigerator for all to see. This chart is for your own personal enjoyment or, better yet, for your own motivation.

If you need scientific accuracy

The Home Fitness Evaluation worksheet is just that: a chart you fill out in your home. I designed it in a simple, non-technical form so that you can get an idea of what your present fitness level is and track your progress in your workout program.

If you want precise scientific measurements, I highly recommend going to a professional for an evaluation. A pro can give you an accurate measurement for each of the tests on this worksheet and will most likely have equipment designed to assess each measurement. When doing your follow-up evaluations, remember to go to the same professional or at least someone who uses the same type of tests and instruments that were used in your first evaluation. This helps to keep all your measurements consistent.

I recommend the following places for a professional fitness evaluation:

- Doctors
- Health clubs
- Health and fitness fairs or expos
- Health or therapy clinics
- Colleges, universities, and YMCAs

Table 8-1 shows you a Home Fitness Evaluation worksheet. Cut it out of the book if you want to make copies for your family and friends to use. Maybe you just want to cut it out so you can hide it under your bed. In either case, I recommend using it. This worksheet is designed to evaluate where your fitness level is now and to help you log your success for the next six months. No, that doesn't mean you can stop working out after six months; you just have to continue your log elsewhere. You never know — someday you may just want to post it up on the refrigerator.

I found a great workout log on the market that I recommend for continuing your exercise diary. *The Ultimate Workout Log* (Houghton Mifflin Co.) by none other than a Dummies author, Suzanne Schlosberg (co-author of *Fitness For Dummies* and *Workouts For Dummies,* IDG Books Worldwide, Inc.).

The Home Fitness Evaluation

I'm not trying to make you a professional fitness evaluator, but I want to give you a good understanding of how to look at and measure yourself objectively and effectively. The numbers for each of the following categories correspond to a section on the Home Fitness Evaluation worksheet (refer to Table 8-1).

Table 8-1	Home Fitness Evaluation Worksheet			

Starting date: _____

	Starting Measure	6 Week Measure	12 Week Measure	24 Week Measure
#1 Resting heart rate				
#2 Target heart rate zone				
#3 Working heart rate				
#4 Total body weight				
#5 Dress size				
#6 Pant size				
#7 Shirt size				
Body fat test:				
#8 Chest (men)				
#9 Abdomen (men & women)				
#10 Triceps (women)				
#11 Thigh (men & women)				
Muscular strength & endurance:				
#12 Push-ups				
#13 Curl-ups				
Flexibility:				
#14 Ceiling stretch				
#15 Cardiovascular test				
Measurements:				
#16 Chest				
#17 Arm				
#18 Waist				
#19 Hip				
#20 Thigh				
#21 Calf				

Determining your resting heart rate (#1)

Your resting heart rate is best measured when you first wake up in the morning, before your feet leave the sheets.

What you need: A stopwatch, or a clock or watch with a second hand

What to do: Find your pulse. You can use two sources to locate the beat. Figure 8-1 demonstrates using the location of your radial artery on your wrist as well as finding your pulse at your carotid artery in your neck.

Choose the spot that works best for you. The only trick to measuring your heart rate is that you must use the correct fingers to do the measuring. Your thumb has a light pulse and can create some confusion when you are counting your beats. It's best to use your index finger and middle finger together (as shown in Figure 8-1).

After you find the beat, you need to count how many beats occur within 60 seconds. The shortcut to this method is to count the number of beats in 10 seconds, and then to multiply that number by 6. This method gives you a 60-second count.

Example: You count 7 beats in 10 seconds: $10 \times 7 = 70$ beats per minute.

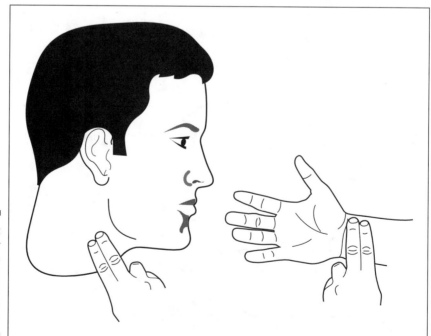

Figure 8-1:
Taking your pulse at the carotid artery and at the radial artery.

Help! If you have trouble finding your pulse or separating the beats in your body from the ticks of your watch, ask a friend for help. Have your friend count your pulse beats while you watch the clock or vice versa.

Your target heart rate zone (#2)

This zone gives you the high and low end for your working heart rate range. The American College of Sports Medicine recommends that your goal should be to attain between 55 to 90 percent of your maximum heart rate when working out. Before you can find your target heart rate zone, you need to figure out your maximum heart rate. To understand some of these heart rate concepts, compare your heart to a car's engine. A car has a tachometer that measures the number of revolutions the engine runs per minute, similar to how many times your heart beats per minute. The red line on a car's tachometer is like a person's maximum heart rate. When the tachometer needle goes past the red line, the car is in danger of combustion. After you figure out where your red line is (your maximum heart rate or the top of your target), you don't want to run your body's engine harder than its limit or above the maximum heart rate.

Note: This formula, although reasonably accurate, may deviate considerably for some people.

What you need: Some math skills or a calculator

What to do: It's easy — just follow the formulas below.

Maximum Heart Rate = 220 minus your age

Example: You are 35 years old. 220 – 35 = 185, your maximum heart rate (MHR)

In order for you to find your target heart rate zone, you need to multiply your maximum heart rate with the low and high zone percentages (55 percent low end and 90 percent high end).

185 (MHR) × .55 = 101.75, the low end of your target heart rate (THR)

185 (MHR) × .90 = 166.50, the high end of your target heart rate (THR)

After you figure out your heart rate goal or zone, mark it in your chart and move on to calculating your working heart rate.

Your working heart rate (#3)

You calculate your working heart rate the same way you found your resting heart rate: by finding your pulse and counting your beats per minute. The difference is that you measure your heart rate while working out. This means you've gotta move your butt, along with a few other body parts, in order to find out how fast your heart is beating while you're exercising.

What you need: A stopwatch; cardiovascular exercise equipment or just your favorite workout outfit and shoes

What to do: Pick a cardiovascular activity like jogging, riding a stationary bike, or using a stair stepper. Get your legs moving for at least 10 to 15 minutes. After you feel like you're working out at a good pace, stop, grab your watch, find your pulse, and start counting.

Example: You are 35 years old. You get on the treadmill, begin your normal jog, and stop after 15 minutes to check your pulse. In 10 seconds you count 25 beats. To find out the 60-second count, you multiply 25 times 6.

25 beats $\times$ 6 = 150, your working heart rate beats per minute

If you look back at the target heart rate zone figured out in the example in #2, you can see you're working out closer to the high end of your zone.

If you don't want to stop your workout to check your heart rate, you can get a heart rate monitor. You can find monitors that strap around your chest or your wrist. If you're interested in purchasing your own heart rate monitor, I recommend the Polar company. Polar offers 10 different models to choose from, and a specialist can help you select the best monitor for your needs. You can speak with a specialist and receive special pricing by contracting Polar at 800-743-9248.

To figure out what percentage of your maximum heart rate you are working out at, simply divide your working heart rate by your maximum heart rate as shown here.

Example: You are 35 years old. Your working heart rate is 150. Your maximum heart rate is 185. 150 ÷ 185 = 81 percent of your maximum heart rate.

Or, to make it easy, use Table 8-2 to find your target heart rate zone. In this table, you see two numbers divided by a slash in each of the percentage columns. The first number is for the working heart rate. The second number is the number of heart beats to count for 10 seconds. You can use the second number if you don't want to do the multiplication to find your working heart rate.

Table 8-2			Target Heart Rate Training Zone Chart			
Age	*80%*	*70%*	*60%*	*Age*	*80%*	*70%*	*60%*
15	164/27	144/24	123/21	19	161/27	141/24	121/20
16	163/27	143/24	122/21	20	160/27	140/23	120/20
17	162/27	142/24	122/21	21	159/27	139/23	119/20
18	162/27	141/24	121/20	22	158/26	139/23	119/20
23	158/26	138/23	118/20	51	135/23	118/20	101/17
24	157/26	137/23	118/20	52	134/22	118/20	101/17
25	156/26	137/23	117/20	53	134/22	117/20	100/17
26	155/26	136/23	116/19	54	133/22	116/19	100/17
27	154/26	135/23	116/19	55	132/22	116/19	99/17
28	154/26	134/22	115/19	56	131/22	115/19	98/16
29	153/26	134/22	115/19	57	130/22	114/19	98/16
30	152/25	133/22	114/19	58	130/22	113/19	97/16
31	151/25	132/22	113/19	59	129/22	113/19	97/16
32	150/25	132/22	113/19	60	128/21	112/19	93/16
33	150/25	131/22	112/19	61	127/21	111/19	95/16
34	149/25	130/22	112/19	62	126/21	111/19	95/16
35	148/25	130/22	111/19	63	126/21	110/18	94/16
36	147/25	129/22	110/18	64	125/21	109/18	94/16
37	146/24	128/21	110/18	65	124/21	108/18	93/16
38	146/24	127/21	109/18	66	123/21	108/18	92/15
39	145/24	127/21	109/18	67	122/20	107/18	92/15
40	144/24	126/21	108/18	68	122/20	106/18	91/15
41	143/24	125/21	107/18	69	121/20	106/18	91/15
42	142/24	124/21	107/18	70	120/20	105/18	90/15
43	142/24	124/21	106/18	71	119/20	104/17	89/15
44	141/24	123/21	106/18	72	118/20	104/17	89/15
45	140/23	123/21	105/18	73	118/20	103/17	88/15
46	139/23	122/20	104/17	74	117/20	102/17	88/15
47	138/23	121/20	104/17	75	116/19	102/17	87/5
48	138/23	120/20	103/17	76	115/19	101/17	86/14
49	137/23	120/20	103/17	77	114/19	100/17	86/14
50	136/23	119/20	102/17	78	114/19	99/17	85/14

Total body weight (#4)

Your weight is easy to measure, but not always pleasant. My advice is *not* to get caught up in your scale weight. This number can be very deceiving. For example, if you have a lot of muscle on your body, your total body weight may seem high. Believe it or not, this is a good thing. The fact is that muscle weighs more than fat. So, in the previous example, a higher body weight may simply indicate that you have a good amount of muscle mass. On the other hand, if you hop on a scale and it reads an attractively low weight, you must consider two options. The first option and best possibility is that you are in great shape and have a balanced fat to muscle ratio. If you haven't done a workout in the past two years, this scenario probably isn't the case. As the other option, your low weight may indicate that you have a high body fat percentage and very little muscle. Remember, fat doesn't weigh as much as muscle, so even though your scale weight is low, you may not be healthy on the inside.

If you have an ectomorph body type (see Chapter 6), you are most likely (if you don't work out) to be the individual who looks skinny on the outside and doesn't weigh much, but who is actually fat on the inside.

Dress, pant, and shirt sizes (#s 5–7)

Different clothing manufacturers seem to have different sizing scales. Have you ever noticed that expensive designer clothes have a slightly smaller scale? For instance, if you are consistently one size for most of your clothes, try on some expensive designer outfit. You may find that a smaller size six actually fits much better. "Yahoo! I got skinny overnight," you think to yourself. Unfortunately, this tactic seems to be a marketing ploy. Consumers are more apt to make a purchase if it makes them feel good about themselves. So when you fill in your chart, pick the dress, pant, and shirt sizes that are most consistent for you.

Body fat measurements (#s 8–11)

The easiest way to get a "guesstimate" of your body fat is to do the Kellogg's cereal "Pinch an Inch" test. Unfortunately, this method doesn't provide you with the most accurate reading of your total body fat, but it is quick and easy. My recommendation is that you have your body fat assessed by a health professional. You can be tested using several different methods, ranging from calipers to hydrostatic weighing (sometimes called water weighing). Testing fees can be anywhere from free to over $100. Find a health professional you like and have him or her do your testing throughout your six-month program evaluation. Being tested using the same method and by the same professional keeps consistency and accuracy in your assessments.

If you just want a general body fat assessment, or if you want to keep this information to yourself, try testing your body fat yourself. One place you can purchase calipers is from the Country Technology corporation. A representative can send you a free catalog and assist you in choosing calipers to do your own personal testing. Prices begin around $35 for a basic pair of calipers (often called *skinfold calipers*). Contact Country Technology at 608-735-4718.

If you decide to try testing your own body fat, follow the directions included with the calipers; then calculate and record your figures on your fitness chart. You can compare your percentages with the standards for men and women listed in Table 8-3.

Table 8-3	Body-Fat Norms	
Classifications	*Women (% fat)*	*Men (% fat)*
Essential fat	11.0–14.0	3.0–5.0
Athletes	12.0–22.0	5.0–13.0
Fitness	16.0–25.0	12.0–18.0
Potential risk	26.0–31.0	19.0–24.0
Obese	32.0+	25.0+

Push yourself up (# 12)

Push-ups, whether they are performed on the toes or knees, are a great way to assess your general *muscle strength*. They are also a good part of an exercise program.

What you need: Just yourself and maybe a partner to count for you

What to do: Get down on all fours and assume the standard hands and toes position or bent-knee position for less intensity and more back support (see Figure 8-2). Without cheating, do as many push-ups as you can until you're exhausted.

Write down the total number of push-ups you did in your Home Fitness Evaluation worksheet. See how well you did by comparing your number with the norms listed in Table 8-4.

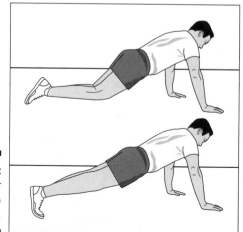

Figure 8-2:
Proper
push-up
form.

Table 8-4	Push-up Norms for Men and Women					
Age (Years)	**(15–19)**		**(20–29)**		**(30–39)**	
Gender	M	F	M	F	M	F
Excellent	≥39	≥33	≥36	≥30	≥30	≥27
Above average	29–38	25–32	29–35	21–29	22–29	20–26
Average	23–28	18–24	22–28	15–20	17–21	13–19
Below average	18–22	12–17	17–21	10–14	12–16	8–12
Poor	≤17	≤11	≤16	≤9	≤11	≤7
Age (Years)	**(40–49)**		**(50–59)**		**(60–69)**	
Gender	M	F	M	F	M	F
Excellent	≥22	≥24	≥21	≥21	≥18	≥17
Above average	17–21	15–23	13–20	11–20	11–17	12–16
Average	13–16	11–14	10–12	7–10	8–10	5–11
Below average	10–12	5–10	7–9	2–6	5–7	1–4
Poor	≤9	≤4	≤6	≤1	≤4	≤1

Abdominal curls (#13)

Doing abdominal curls, which is one of the best ways to tighten your abdominals, is also a good method for checking your *muscle endurance*.

What you need: Yourself and, if you choose, a partner to count for you and hold your feet to the floor.

What to do: Lie down on your back with your knees bent. Have your partner hold your feet to the floor or place your toes under a couch. Place your hands behind your head and keep your chin off your chest. Lift your chest toward the ceiling and then lower yourself back down to the floor (repeatedly) until you reach exhaustion (see Figure 8-3).

Write your total on your chart and compare it with the chart in Table 8-5.

Table 8-5	Sit-up Norms for Men and Women					
Category	**Number Completed**					
	Men/Age			**Women/Age**		
	<35	35–44	>45	<35	35–44	>45
Excellent	60	50	40	50	40	30
Good	45	40	25	40	30	15
Marginal	30	25	15	25	15	10
Needs work	15	10	5	10	6	4

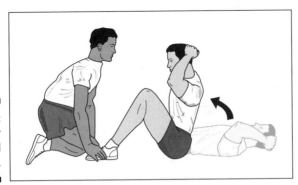

Figure 8-3: Proper abdominal curl form.

Stretching to the ceiling (#14)

Your ability to extend your hamstrings (see Chapter 13 for more information on leg muscles) is a good indicator of your spine, hip, and hamstring flexibility.

What you need: A mat, or something comfortable to lie on, and a partner or a mirror if you need help in determining your maximum stretch.

What to do: Lie on your back with one leg lying on the floor. Raise the opposite leg up towards the ceiling by placing your hands behind your knee (for a better grip, interlock your fingertips). With your hands, pull your leg in towards your chest, keeping your knee as straight as possible and your foot flexed (pull your toes towards your nose). A measurement of good flexibility would be 80° to 90° of hip flexion. This means that your leg would be perpendicular (at a right angle) to the floor. Figure 8-4 demonstrates this flexibility test and gives you a better perspective of the angle measurement. In general, you can assess your flexibility by gauging it on the following:

Greater than 80 to 90 degrees of hip flexion = Excellent flexibility

Equal to 80 to 90 degrees of hip flexion = Good flexibility

Less than 80 to 90 degrees of hip flexion = Below average flexibility

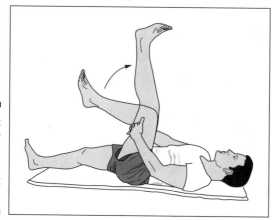

Figure 8-4:
Proper ceiling stretch measurement form.

Determining your cardiovascular fitness (#15)

The step test is an easy way to calculate your cardiovascular fitness.

What you need: A box or a step, a stopwatch or a clock with a second hand, and a partner to help you time the test

What to do: First locate your pulse as described in the section on resting heart rate (#1). Now, start stepping up and down for 3 minutes (as shown in Figure 8-5).

As soon as you're done, find your pulse again and record the number of beats per minute. Remember from the resting heart rate test that you can count your beats for 10 seconds and multiply that number by 6 to get the total number of beats per minute. Check your fitness level in the chart in Table 8-6.

Table 8-6	Cardiovascular Step Test Pulse Rate Tables for Men and Women			
Fitness Level	*18–29 Years*		*30–57 Years*	
	Men	*Women*	*Men*	*Women*
Excellent	69–75	76–84	63–75	73–86
Good	76–83	85–94	77–90	87–100
Average	84–92	95–105	91–106	101–116
Fair	93–99	106–116	107–120	117–130
Poor	100–106	117–127	121–134	131–144

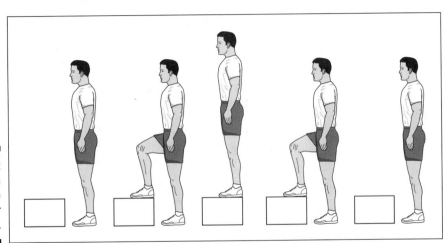

Figure 8-5: Proper form for the cardiovascular step test.

Taking your measurements (#s 16–21)

It's time to break out the measuring tape and strip down to your underwear. You may want to do these measurements yourself. If you're feeling pretty confident or if you're an exhibitionist, you can ask a partner to help you out.

What you need: A measuring tape

What to do: Measure the location points for each part of the body that I ask you to measure. Check out Figure 8-6 for precise locations.

  ✔ **#16 Chest:** Place the measuring tape along the nipple line.

  ✔ **#17 Arm:** The tape should cover the upper arm just below the armpit.

  ✔ **#18 Waist:** Find your narrowest point and wrap the tape around it.

  ✔ **#19 Hips:** (Women only) Slide the tape up and down to find your widest point and measure away.

  ✔ **#20 Thighs:** Look for the widest point in your thigh (upper leg) and measure.

  ✔ **#21 Calf:** This one isn't ego damaging unless you're a guy with really skinny calves. Some guys may want to contract their calves before searching for the widest point to measure.

To Be Conditioned, or Not to Be

After you evaluate your fitness level, you can determine the level of your initial workout program. Review numbers 12, 13, 14, and 15 on your worksheet and compare your scores for these tests with the accompanying charts I provide earlier in the chapter. Note which category you fall under for each test (good, average, poor, and so on). If your scores fall in ranges labeled fair, marginal, needs work, below average, or poor, place yourself in the *deconditioned category*. Any scores above these levels put you in the *conditioned category*. Another way to assess your conditioning is the Couch Potato Test. If you spend more time on the couch than you do moving around, you probably want to start off in the deconditioned category. The following categories give you the format for your own exercise program based on your conditioning. If you're starting off with the deconditioned workout routine, stick with it for your first six weeks. If you feel pretty good and your test scores improve on your second evaluation, give yourself a big star, put your scores up on the fridge, and move yourself into the conditioned category.

You can find your personal *Exercise Program Chart* in Appendix A. If you want to make copies before you fill in your chart, cut along the dotted line. After you choose your workout routine, follow the steps to fill out your chart and keep it handy for your workouts.

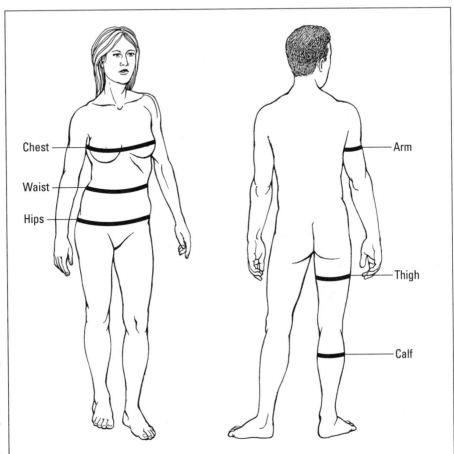

Figure 8-6:
Precise
locations
for body
measurements.

Deconditioned workout routine

Step 1: Selecting your favorite exercises

Select 1 to 2 exercises *per* muscle group. You can choose the exercises
located on your *Exercise Program Chart* in Appendix A (which are covered in
Chapters 9 through 18), or fill in some of your own exercises in the blank
spaces provided.

Step 2: Sets and repetitions

The American College of Sports Medicine, based on the findings of 35
studies in the literature, recommends 1 *set* (a group of consecutive repetitions) per weight training exercise reaching the maximum intensity for the
entire set. Personally I have found that most of my deconditioned clientele
receive greater benefits without any negative effects by performing 2 sets of

ADVANCED STUFF

The highs and lows of weights and repetitions

In the spectrum of resistance training, from high weights and low repetitions to low weights and high repetitions, you get different results depending on the way you perform your exercises. True, lifting heavy weights will make your muscles larger, but it doesn't do you much good if you can't do anything but look in the mirror and flex. Then again, if all you do is high-repetition exercises, you're not going to develop much muscularity. If you've been body watching long enough, you may be able to tell what type of workout someone does based on his or her muscular development. For example, most bodybuilders utilize heavy weights, incorporating power exercises such as squats and military presses to bulk up their bodies during the off season. Then they increase the repetitions of each exercise, reduce the amount of weight they are lifting, and begin aerobic type exercises in order to *cut up*

(improve definition) for the next competition. On the other hand, check out competitive cyclists or runners. Their muscles tend to be less bulky, but more lean and defined.

When you're setting personal goals, look at the bodies of competitive athletes and see which muscle types appeal to you. Before selecting your role model, check to see what body type you have and what type your model has (see Chapters 5, 6, and 7). Remember: If you are 5 feet 2 inches tall (1.6 meters) and weigh 125 pounds (57 kg), don't hope for Michael Jordan's physique. No workout can help you with that goal. If you have a physique that's even somewhat similar to your role model's, you can emulate his or her workouts on a smaller scale, which may (in part) help you achieve your goals.

each exercise. You choose the guideline, which suits your personal needs, but remember your goal is eventually to be able to increase the intensity and duration of your workouts. Each set should contain 8 to 10 repetitions or reps (the number of times you perform the exercise).

Example: Exercise: Biceps curl
Repetitions: 8 to 10
Sets: 2

Step 3: How much weight

To determine how much weight you should use when performing your exercises, refer to Chapters 9 through 18. I give a dumbbell size recommendation for each exercise listed. In general, the best way to select weights is to start light and work your way up. If you can perform all the repetitions for each set of a particular exercise, you should increase the weight you are using. It is normal to experience muscle fatigue during the last few repetitions of your last set. This fatigue is an indication you are getting the most out of your exercise.

Stimulate your muscles

The propulsion mechanism common to all mammals is skeletal muscle. Skeletal muscle is made up of thousands, even millions, of tiny units that have the ability to contract. These units are called *myofibrils*. The greater the number of these myofibrils, the bigger the muscle and hence the stronger the muscle.

Your muscles have the ability to generate new and greater numbers of myofibrils when stimulated correctly. Stressing a muscle by resistance training forces the muscle to adapt by producing more myofibrils. In addition, increasing the resistance with heavier weights generally stimulates even greater numbers of myofibrils, leading to bulkier muscles. In contrast, using lighter weights with higher repetitions forces the muscle to adapt by utilizing its energy more efficiently. A combination of training, called cross-training (not cross-dressing), continually stimulates your muscles, not only enlarging them, but also keeping them in better aerobic shape.

Step 4: Cardiovascular exercise

The U.S. Surgeon General issued a report in July of 1997 recommending 30 minutes of moderate exercise per day. Although this may include activities such as walking to work, gardening, or walking up stairs, I recommend you focus your cardiovascular workouts on more intense activities such as walking briskly or swimming for 30 minutes. If you feel good and you reach your target heart rate zone (see #2 earlier in the chapter), increase your duration. You'll increase your caloric expenditure and see the results sooner!

Conditioned workout routine

Step 1: Selecting your favorite exercises

Although the American College of Sports Medicine states that a conditioned individual will receive benefits from performing 1 set of 8 to 10 repetitions (of maximum intensity), I feel in order to significantly improve your level of fitness you should select 2 to 3 exercises *per* muscle group. You can choose the exercises located on your *Exercise Program Chart* in Appendix A (which are covered in Chapters 9 through 18), or fill in some exercises of your own in the blank spaces provided.

LINGO

Be a bully: Pull and push your weight around

As you perform muscle-conditioning exercises, you'll begin to notice that you are usually pulling and pushing your weight around. In other words, you're flexing and extending your skeletal muscles. For example, the muscle group in the front of your thigh is called the quadriceps. These muscles control the movement of your knee, causing it to extend and straighten your leg. (Think of kicking a ball.) In this movement you extend, or push, your foot forward in order to straighten your leg and make contact with the ball.

When one muscle group extends, the opposing muscle group should flex. In this case, the opposing muscle group consists of the hamstrings, which are located in the back of your thigh. The hamstring muscles, like the quadriceps, work to move your knee, but this group flexes, or pulls, your foot toward your buns.

This figure shows you the skeletal muscles for which you can find exercises in Chapters 10–20. Each one has a specific movement as you perform the exercise. Knowing what your muscles are created to do gives you a better understanding of the exercises I've listed for you. You'll also be able to find other exercises to work your muscles by knowing what their movements are.

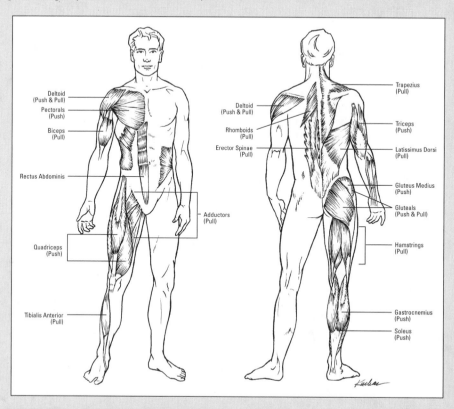

Step 2: Sets and repetitions

Perform 3 sets (a group of consecutive repetitions) of each exercise you choose. Each set should contain 10 to 12 repetitions or reps (the number of times you perform the exercise).

Example: Exercise: Biceps curl
Repetitions: 10 to 12
Sets: 3

Step 3: How much weight

To determine how much weight you should use when performing your exercises, refer to Chapters 9 through 18. I give a dumbbell size recommendation for each exercise listed. In general, the best way to select weights is to start light and work your way up. If you can perform all the repetitions for each set of a particular exercise, you should increase the weight you are using. It is normal to experience muscle fatigue during the last few repetitions of your last set. This fatigue is an indication you are getting the most out of your exercise.

Step 4: Cardiovascular exercise

Perform your chosen cardio activity for a 30- to 45-minute duration. If you feel good and you reach your target heart rate zone (see #2 earlier in the chapter), increase your duration. You will increase your caloric expenditure and see the results sooner.

Variety is the key to maintaining the motivation to work out. Change your program every six weeks or as often as you like. You can select different muscle-toning exercises or cardio activities to best suit your needs, your enjoyment, or your time schedule. As your muscle strength and endurance increase, your exercise duration or frequency, and the weight resistance you use or the intensity of your workout, should also increase.

Part III
Upper-Body Workouts

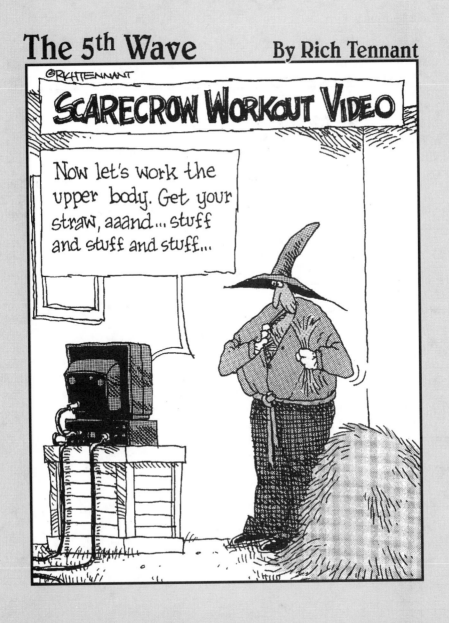

The 5th Wave   By Rich Tennant

SCARECROW WORKOUT VIDEO

Now let's work the upper body. Get your straw, aaand... stuff and stuff and stuff...

In this part . . .

1 t's time to get your heart and upper-body muscles moving. I give you tips on choosing cardiovascular exercises and the best exercises for burning calories. I list a variety of my favorite upper-body muscle-conditioning exercises so that you can start pumping up your arms, chest, back, and abdominals. You can pick from the exercises I list and also choose your own favorites to put in your personal workout program.

Chapter 9

Cardiovascular Exercise

● ●

In This Chapter

▶ Revving up your heart

▶ Burning calories

▶ Choosing your cardiovascular activities

● ●

*W*hy should you do cardiovascular exercise? Because your heart is your most valuable muscle! Your body is a machine and your heart is its engine. Just like an automobile, your body needs quality fuel (which translates to low-fat, nutritious foods), and regular checkups to keep the engine in good condition.

The heart is an incredibly complex organ; however, it is also a muscle. It just happens to have valves and blood flowing through it. Just like any other muscle, if you don't work it, it's going to atrophy (that means become a flabby mess). Unlike the muscles of your arms and legs, your heart gets its workout from beating quickly for prolonged periods at a time. The heart responds to the metabolic demands of your muscles. So when you're exercising and contracting your muscles in prolonged activities such as swimming, jogging, or cycling, you're exercising your heart.

ADVANCED STUFF

Metabolic fitness

Many new studies show that lack of exercise and an increase of fat in your daily diet lead to *metabolic syndrome* in adults, which manifests itself as insulin resistance and a high level of insulin. These conditions inevitably cause health risks such as hypertension, obesity, increased cholesterol, decreased levels of HDL, and artery-clotting abnormalities.

Revving Up the Engine Muscle

By performing cardiovascular (or cardio, for short) activities, you increase the strength of your heart muscle. The benefits of *cardiorespiratory endurance exercises* (activities that primarily exercise your heart) are numerous. For example, by regularly exercising your most vital muscle you can:

- ✔ Relieve stress and body tension.
- ✔ Increase your overall energy.
- ✔ Burn calories and body fat, and increase or maintain lean body mass.
- ✔ Reduce the risk of some cancers.
- ✔ Prevent osteoporosis.
- ✔ Lower your blood pressure.
- ✔ Reduce the risk of heart disease.
- ✔ Improve your body's metabolic efficiency.
- ✔ Improve your ability to exercise in hot weather.
- ✔ Live longer.

The impact of it all

Have you ever wondered what those silly aerobic schedules mean when they describe their classes as high or low impact? Well, there is a difference. *High-impact* movement occurs when both feet simultaneously lose contact with the ground. *Low-impact* movement occurs when one or both feet are consistently in contact with the ground.

Just like aerobic dance, various cardiovascular activities can be labeled high or low impact. See Table 9-1 for a breakdown of high- and low-impact cardiovascular activities.

Table 9-1	High- and Low-Impact Cardiovascular Activities
High Impact	**Low Impact**
Running	Walking
Jogging	Swimming
Jumping rope	Bicycling

High Impact	Low Impact
Fast tempo aerobic dance	In-line or ice skating
	Slow tempo aerobic dance
	Skiing (no moguls)
	Stair climbing

Determining if one activity is better than another really depends on you. If you experience lower-back pain or any joint pain while taking a brisk walk, then high-impact activities aren't going to help your aches and pains. In fact, they will probably increase your pain. On the other hand, if you have no joint or back pain during or after a run, you can probably perform other high-impact activities without discomfort. The key word I want you to note is *pain*. Many people don't listen to their bodies, and at the end of a workout, they have more pain than when they started. See Chapter 4 for more information on injury prevention.

Your body weight is what you're working with as a form of resistance. If your weight is 135 pounds (61.2 kg), you have 135 pounds of resistance in your movements. Your bones and joints absorb that impact as you perform the exercise. If you are overweight, that extra weight actually increases your chance of injury. If you're not sure what type of impact is best for you, start out low and work your way up. Try a brisk walk and assess how your body feels afterward. If you feel like the Energizer Bunny, pick up your pace and move into an easy jog or run. Whatever form of cardio exercise you choose, be smart about it. Ask yourself a few questions before you sign yourself up for the next Iron Man or Woman Triathlon.

- How far do you feel you can run, comfortably? Is your body ready to run a marathon?
- Can you glide through the water or do you sink?
- Are you coordinated enough to do all those moves in an aerobic dance class, or do you go one way when everyone else is going another?

Keep in mind that whether you choose high- or low-impact activities, your body needs some type of cardio workout. You want to feel good during and after your workout, so choose wisely.

The keys to cardio exercise are:

- **Movement:** You gotta move your body.
- **Legs:** Legs are your primary movers. Movement of the big muscle groups of your lower body helps to get your heart pumping.

The goal of cardio exercise is to get your heart pumping and into your target heart rate zone (see Chapter 8 for more on calculating your target heart rate zone). After you have achieved your target heart rate, try and maintain it for 30 minutes or longer if you can.

Know your body. A quick, easy way to see if you're working within your target heart rate while doing cardio exercise is to check your *rate of perceived exertion*. This rating has no formula because it is based on how your whole body *feels* — your lungs, heart, muscles, and so on. If you can keep moving and recite your phone number, address, and credit card number, stop for a moment, write it down, and mail it to me. Just kidding! What you really need to do is to determine how you feel. If you can talk to yourself or your fitness partner without having to gasp for air in between each word, and your partner can understand you pretty well, you're probably doing okay. If you can't speak to your partner and feel like you're ready to pass out, you definitely want to slow down your pace.

Another way to measure your perceived exertion is to rate your level of internal and external fatigue on a scale of 0 to 10. Look at the example quotes I've listed and see where are you on that scale. Table 9-2 is a general guide to your rate of perceived exertion. You may find yourself right in line with the three levels listed or somewhere in between.

Table 9-2	Rate of Perceived Exertion	
Numeric Rating	*Level of Difficulty Rating*	*How Do You Feel?*
0	No difficulty	"I could do this all day long."
5	Somewhat hard	"This is getting hard, but I can go a bit longer."
10	Very, very hard	"Oh my! I think I'm dying!"

Moving muscles, burning calories

So you want to move some muscle and burn some calories? Different activities require the use of different muscle groups. Table 9-3 is a list of exercises and activities that require cardiovascular resistance and muscle strength and endurance. Although any exercise helps your body burn calories, the activities checked off in the cardio column are the most effective for burning fat and calories. As you can see, most of the activities require the strength and endurance of most of your major muscle groups. The number of stars in each column tells you the degree to which that muscle group is used. The more stars listed in the column, the greater the need for muscle strength and endurance in a particular area. If you know which muscles are your best assets, you can select an activity that best suits you. If you want to improve strength in certain parts of your body, look for an activity that helps you develop those muscles. Focusing part of your exercise routine on building up specific muscle groups can help you improve your performance in the sport of your choice.

Table 9-3	Muscle Activity in Cardio Exercise						
Activity	**Cardio Exercise**	**Back**	**Shoulders**	**Arms**	**Abdomen**	**Hips**	**Legs**
Baseball		*	*	*	*	*	*
Basketball	**	*	*	*	*	*	***
Boxing	**	**	**	***	**	*	***
Cross-country running	***	*	*	*	*	*	***
Fencing	*	*	*	*	*	*	**
Gymnastics (floor exercise)		*	*	***	*	*	**
Field hockey	**	*	*	*	*	*	***
Ice hockey	**	*	*	*	*	*	*
Judo	*	**	**	***	**	*	***
Karate	*	**	**	***	**	*	***
Rugby	**		*	*			***
Soccer	**	*			*	*	***
Swimming	**	**	*	***	**	*	***
Tennis	**	*	*	*	*	*	***
Water polo	**	*	*	**	*	*	*
Waterskiing	*	*	*	**	*		**
Weight lifting		**	**	**	**	**	**
Wrestling	*	**	*	***	**	*	*

Burning calories

I know what you're thinking: "That information is just fine and dandy, but how many calories can I really burn?" Calories seem to be something we're eating all day long and forever trying to burn off, yet many of us don't even know what they are.

Energy and calories

Energy is measured by calories. You call a unit of measure a large calorie or a kilocalorie (kcal), which is equal to 1,000 small calories. Calorie and kcal are often used interchangeably, by the way. A kilocalorie is the amount of heat required to raise 1 kilogram of water 1 degree Celsius.

Three major nutrients are in a calorie: carbohydrates, proteins, and fat (which is called the "fuel factor"). The fuel factor helps you understand the nutrition information listed on the foods you purchase. Each fuel factor consists of:

1 gram of carbohydrate = 4 calories

1 gram of protein = 4 calories

1 gram of fat = 9 calories

To better understand this formula, look at the following example. If you purchase a food that has:

20 grams of carbs, 6 grams of protein, and 4 grams of fat, the total caloric value of that food is 140 calories. Great math skills aren't necessary to figure out how I came up with the answer.

20 g x 4 cal. each gram = 80 calories from carbohydrates

6 g x 4 cal. each gram = 24 calories from protein

4 g x 9 cal. each gram = 36 calories from fat

You get these fuel factors through the foods you eat and convert them into energy units of glucose (sugar) that are burned in order to release energy. If you don't use them, you store them in the form of fat. Your body converts these fuel factors by your metabolism, which is the chemical reaction of a cell that transfers unusable materials into energy. This energy is used for your body's activities (brain and nerve activity, muscle contraction, and the regulation of your body temperature).

As you move, your body releases energy in the form of heat. That's why your body sweats when you work out — to release this heat to regulate your core temperature. You need food for your body to survive, yet you need to exercise your body to release the extra calories you eat every day.

Pick your favorite activities from Table 9-4 and start calculating. Find the weight closest to yours and match it up with your selected exercise to determine total calories burned per hour.

I list the average amount of calories burned if you are performing the activity for an hour. The key word is *average*. I can't make promises, because it's up to you to work to the best of your ability.

Table 9-4	How Many Calories Am I Burning?		
Activity	*kcal/hour*	*kcal/hour*	*kcal/hour*
	110 lbs	*154 lbs*	*198 lbs*
Archery	150–200	210–280	270–360
Backpacking	250–550	350–770	450–990
Badminton	200–450	280–630	360–810
Basketball	150–600	210–840	270–1080
Billiards	125	175	225
Bowling	100–200	140–280	180–360
Boxing	400–650	560–910	720–1170
Canoeing/Rowing/ Kayaking	150–400	210–560	270–720
Cricket	200–350	280–490	360–630
Croquet	175	245	315
Cycling	150–400+	210–560+	270–720+
Dancing: social/tap	150–350	210–490	270–630
Dancing: aerobic	200–500	280–700	360–900
Fencing	300–500	420–700	540–900
Field hockey	400	560	720
Fishing	100–200	140–280	180–360
Football (touch)	300–500	420–700	540–900
Golf: with cart	100–150	140–210	180–270
Golf: pulling clubs	200–350	280–490	270–630
Handball	400–600	560–480	720–1080
Hiking	260–350	210–490	270–360
Horseback riding	150–400	210–560	270–720
Horseshoe pitching	100–150	140–210	180–270
Hunting: bow or gun	150–350	210–490	270–630
Jogging	535	750	960
Paddleball/Racquetball	400–600	560–840	720–1080
Rope jumping	450–600	630–810	810–1080
Running	765	1070	1380
Sailing	100–250	140–350	180–450

(continued)

Table 9-4 *(continued)*

Activity	kcal/hour 110 lbs	kcal/hour 154 lbs	kcal/hour 198 lbs
Scuba diving	250–500	350–700	450–900
Shuffleboard	100–150	140–210	180–270
Skating: ice or roller	250–400	350–560	450–720
Skiing: downhill	250–400	350–560	450–720
Skiing: cross country	300–600	420–840	540–1080
Skiing: water	250–350	350–490	450–630
Sledding	200–400	280–560	360–720
Snowshoeing	350–700	490–980	630–1260
Squash	400–600	560–840	720–1080
Soccer	250–600	350–840	450–1080
Swimming	430	600	770
Table tennis	150–250	210–350	270–450
Tennis	200–450	280–630	360–810
Volleyball	150–300	210–420	270–540

ADVANCED STUFF

The yellow jacket

The *yellow jacket* is a plastic surgery term for the subcutaneous fatty layer that surrounds your body just under your skin. Your body's fat is a repository of stored energy that is utilized by your organs and muscles as fuel. The energy utilization of your organs, however, remains relatively low versus the utilization of your muscles, which use up to a thousand-fold more energy during intense activity. The more muscle mass you have, the more fuel you burn each time you work out. In addition, while you're at rest, your muscles, which are metabolically active (especially if they're growing in response to resistance training), continue to burn fat. Many athletes can eat just about whatever they want and not pile on the pounds because of their high percentages of muscle mass. The bottom line is that if you eat low-fat, healthy foods and perform resistance training exercises regularly, your yellow jacket will melt away. Add aerobic exercise to your program and you'll never have to worry about liposuction.

As you can see, when you increase your muscle mass, your body works harder and exerts more energy in all your daily activities. This increased energy output means that you are burning more calories than when you had less muscle mass. The end result . . . you lose fat both by decreasing your overall body fat and increasing your muscle mass.

Let's Get Moving

Although Table 9-4 lists many different activities you may participate in, I picked a few of the most popular cardio exercises to offer you hints on how best to perform them. Before you get started with any of these activities, make sure you warm up and stretch out (see Chapter 3 for examples) and are equipped with the appropriate shoes, clothes, and any safety gear needed (see Chapter 2 for tips on the right gear). In addition, I include some cool programs for walking, jogging, biking, and swimming. Cut them out, make copies, and get your body moving!

Walking

Walking is a great way to initiate an exercise program. It's a popular activity because it's convenient and is a natural movement. You can take a walk in your neighborhood, at the beach, on a nature trail, or on a treadmill. People who are obese or have a great deal of joint pain should choose walking as one of their primary exercises.

Start your walking program with a light stretch (see Chapter 3); then start walking at a slow speed and pick up your pace when you feel comfortable. As you pick up your pace, remember to breathe through your nose and mouth. You can build your program by increasing your speed, distance, or both.

Keep in mind the following tips on correct body form:

- ✔ Keep the trunk of your body upright, with a slight arch in your lower back, and keep your chest and chin up.
- ✔ Take strides that feel comfortable to you and keep your feet pointed forward.
- ✔ Your feet should contact the ground in a heel to toe direction.
- ✔ Let your arms swing back and forth freely, which helps you keep your balance, increase your heart rate, and burn more calories.

See Table 9-5 to create your own walking program. Take it at your own pace, but try to exercise at one stage per week. For example, you initiate your walking program with Stage 1 on the chart. You decide to walk 3 times per week and stay at Stage 1 for the first week. The second week of your program you move up to Stage 2 of the program. Each week you advance to the next stage and continually record your heart rate (see Chapter 8) and how you feel.

Table 9-5		Walking Program	
Stage	*Duration*	*Heart rate*	*Comments*
1	15 min		
2	20 min		
3	25 min		
4	30 min		
5	30 min		
6	30 min		
7	35 min		
8	40 min		
9	45 min		
10	45 min		
11	45 min		
12	50 min		
13	55 min		
14	60 min		
15	60 min		
16	60 min		
17	60 min		
18	60 min		
19	60 min		
20	60 min		

Reprinted by permission from Franks, B. and E. Howley, 1989, *Fitness Leader's Handbook,* (Champaign, IL: Human Kinetics), 265.

Jogging

Picking up the pace in your walk may lead you into a slow jog. If this feels comfortable to you and you have the appropriate shoes on, go for it (see Chapter 3 for more on the proper equipment). The warm-up and body form tips are the same for jogging as for walking, but the overall intensity of the movement increases. You may notice that your movements become high impact due to your increased speed. Exaggerate your arm swing to keep up with the pace your legs are setting.

Table 9-6 provides you with a progressive jogging program. I recommend you progress through and past the walking program before starting to jog. Keep a journal of how you feel after each jog or each week to show your progress and results.

Table 9-6	Jogging Program	
Stage	**Description**	**How do you feel?**
1	Jog 10 steps, walk 10 steps. Repeat 5 times and take your heart rate. Stay within your Target Heart Rate (THR) zone by increasing or decreasing walking phase. Do 20 to 30 minutes of activity.	
2	Jog 20 steps, walk 10 steps. Repeat 5 times and take your heart rate. Stay within your THR zone by increasing or decreasing walking phase. Do 20 to 30 minutes of activity.	
3	Jog 30 steps, walk 10 steps. Repeat 5 times and take your heart rate. Stay within your THR zone by increasing or decreasing walking phase. Do 20 to 30 minutes of activity.	
4	Jog 1 minute, walk 10 steps. Repeat 3 times and take your heart rate. Stay within your THR zone by increasing or decreasing walking phase. Do 20 to 30 minutes of activity.	
5	Jog 2 minutes, walk 10 steps. Repeat 2 times and take your heart rate. Stay within your THR zone by increasing or decreasing walking phase. Do 30 minutes of activity.	
6	Jog 1 lap on a track (400 m or 440 yd) and check your heart rate. Adjust pace during run to stay within the THR zone. If heart rate is still too high, go back to the Stage 5 schedule. Do 6 laps with a brief walk between each.	
7	Jog 2 laps and check heart rate. Adjust pace during run to stay within the THR zone. If heart rate is still too high, go back to the Stage 6 activity. Do 6 laps with a brief walk between each.	
8	Jog 1 mile (1.6 km) and check heart rate. Adjust pace during run to stay within the THR zone. Do 2 miles.	
9	Jog 2 to 3 miles (3.2 to 4.8 km) continuously. Check heart rate at the end to ensure that you were within the THR zone.	

Reprinted by permission from Franks, B. and E. Howley, 1989, *Fitness Leader's Handbook*, (Champaign, IL: Human Kinetics), 266.

Bicycling

Biking is a great form of cardio exercise and is a lot of fun whether you are on the road, in the mountains, or on a stationary bike. If you're looking for a low-impact, minimal weight-bearing activity, cycling is one of your best choices. Table 9-7 provides you with a progressive cycling program.

Riding a bike doesn't have as much impact on your lower-body joints as jogging or running do, but I still caution those of you who have knee injuries or back problems to check with your doctor before starting a cycling program.

Spinning classes are the newest craze in fitness centers across the country. The class members (and you) are provided with a stationary bike, and the instructor takes you through an intense workout. If you're into cycling I highly recommend trying out a spinning class. You can read more about spinning in Chapter 21.

As always, I recommend a warm-up and a stretch before starting your workout. (See Chapter 3 for details on warming up and stretching.) Many stationary bikes have warm-ups programmed into them, but if you are biking outdoors, spend the first 3 to 5 minutes of your ride warming up your muscles. Although you may feel like you can bike forever, it's not advisable to jump on your bike and immediately head for the hills.

If you choose a stationary bike, try the electronic workout programs it offers. The electronic workouts can vary from gradually increasing intensity to random bouts of hilly terrain. Your other option is a road or mountain bike. You may want to get a safety check and tune up before you hit the road to prevent any unwanted injuries or collisions.

If you decide to bike outdoors for cardio exercise, you need to keep your heart rate elevated in your target heart rate zone (see Chapter 8). The best way to accomplish this is to pick a course with as few stops as possible, and maybe attempt a hill or two during your ride. You can't count a casual ride around the neighborhood, stopping every few miles to talk with a neighbor, look in a store window, or grab an ice cream cone, as an intense cardiovascular workout.

Follow this list of tips for body form when you cycle:

- Adjust your seat level before you begin riding. When you are seated on the bike and have one leg fully extended, you should have a slight bend in your knee. A good way to measure this is to place one pedal in the bottom position of its rotation. With your heel on the pedal, your knee should be almost straight.

✔ When you are ready to begin, place the ball of your foot on the pedal. You should have a slight bend in your knees as they move through the rotation.

✔ The trunk of your body should be inclined forward and the handlebars should be at least as high as your seat.

✔ Your wrists should be mostly straight with no excessive bend forward or backward.

Table 9-7	Biking Program	
Stage	**Description**	**How Do You Feel?**
1	Find a bike path or roads you feel comfortable riding on. Begin stage one biking on a flat surface with minimal or no hills. Keep pedaling at a comfortable level of resistance for 20 to 30 minutes.	
2	At stage two, add in a few biking sprints. Bike at a normal, cardiovascularly comfortable pace for 10 minutes, and then pedal as fast as you can for 2 minutes. Repeat the 10 minute/ 2 minute pattern 2 or 3 times. Check your heart rate after your sprint to make sure you're not exceeding your maximum heart rate.	
3	Now that you're able to bring your heart rate up and down, try to increase the difficulty and the duration of your program. Begin with your comfortable pace (which may be a bit more intense at this point or at a more difficult speed) and continue it for 15 to 20 minutes. If you have a hill you can bike up, try it. If not, increase the intensity of your speed and the resistance of your pedaling for 5 minutes. Follow this pattern 2 or 3 times. Concentrate on using your legs and buns to help you up any hills. Check your heart rate or rate of perceived exertion (see Chapter 8) and try to stay within your THR zone.	

(continued)

Table 9-7 *(continued)*

Stage	Description	How Do You Feel?
4	Create your own pedaling course. Make your overall goal to increase the duration of your overall biking time and increase the amount of resistance you're pedaling with (use higher gears on the bike). Attempting to climb uphill helps develop your lower body muscles, and you burn more calories as you increase the overall amount of time on your ride. At this stage you should be able to ride for 30 to 60 minutes with at least 2 to 4 sprints, or a ride up a hill.	

Swimming

Finding a pool, lake, or ocean may not be as easy as finding a bike or place to walk, but swimming is still an option to consider. You may find a place to swim at your local community center, YMCA, or YWCA. If you find a location, I recommend that you give swimming a try. Swimming is a no-impact activity and a great way to work your heart, lungs, and almost every muscle in your body. Many physical therapists recommend swimming to their patients who have injuries and therefore find it difficult to walk or ride a bike.

If you don't know how to swim or you want to learn new strokes, take some lessons. Another option is to try the swimming program I include for you in Table 9-8. You may even want to check out a water aerobics class. Whatever form of exercise you choose in the pool, remember to warm up, stretch (see Chapter 3), and start your program at your own pace. Take breaks to check your heart rate and keep yourself within your target heart rate zone (see Chapter 8). You may even want to grab a mask, a snorkel, goggles, or floating devices to make you feel more comfortable if you aren't used to being in the water. The best way to learn proper body form in the water is to take a lesson. Check out your local YMCA or gym to see if they offer any programs.

Table 9-8 offers you a water cardio endurance workout that you can walk or jog. Follow the stages and keep track of your progress in a journal or on your swimming program chart.

Table 9-8	Swimming Program	
Stage	*Description*	*How Do You Feel?*
1	In chest-deep water, walk across the width of the pool 4 times and see if you are close to your Target Heart Rate (THR). Gradually increase the duration of the walk until you can do 2 10-minute walks at THR.	
2	In chest-deep water, walk across and jog back. Repeat 2 times and see if you are close to THR. Gradually increase the duration of the jogging until you can do 4 5-minute jogs at THR.	
3	In chest-deep water, walk across and swim back (any stroke). Use kickboard or flotation device if needed. Repeat this cycle 2 times and see if you are at THR. Keep up this pattern of walk-swim to do about 20 to 30 minutes of activity.	
4	In chest-deep water, jog across and swim back (any stroke); repeat and check THR. Gradually decrease the duration of the jog and increase the duration of the swim until you can complete 4 widths within the THR zone. Accomplish 20 to 30 minutes of activity per session.	
5	Slowly swim 25 yards (22.9 m), rest 30 seconds, slowly swim another 25 yards, and check THR. On the basis of the heart rate response, change the speed of the swim and/or the length of the rest period to stay within the THR zone. Gradually increase the number of lengths you can swim (3, then 4, and so on) before checking THR.	
6	Increase the duration of continuous swimming until you can accomplish 20 to 30 minutes without a rest.	

Reprinted by permission from Franks, B. and E. Howley, 1989, *Fitness Leader's Handbook*, (Champaign, IL: Human Kinetics), 271.

Quick calorie burners

If you don't have time for your regular cardio-vascular workout, these suggestions help you to keep your feet moving and your heart pumping.

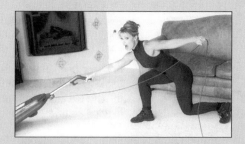

- ✔ Walk your dog, your baby, your friend, or yourself.

- ✔ Find some stairs and start climbing. If you're feeling lucky, try climbing two or three at a time.

- ✔ Put on your favorite music and start dancing. You may find out you have a new talent.

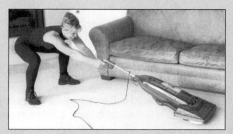

- ✔ Sweep the floors, vacuum, or mow the lawn. These may not be the most exciting activities, but they do burn calories.

The bottom line is that you've gotta move your body. Sitting on the couch waiting for your muscles to get in shape just doesn't work. We all wish it did, but no such luck. So get up and move. You'll feel better, look better, and find even more ways to enjoy life.

Chapter 10

Flex Your Pecs: Arm and Chest Exercises

. . . .

In This Chapter

▶ Working your chest and arm muscles

▶ Determining your sets and repetitions

▶ Avoiding mistakes while exercising your chest and arms

. . . .

*P*opeye had a great idea when he picked spinach as a food to help him build muscle and strength. Nutritional foods may start you on your way to a healthier body, but it's going to take a little more than spinach to build those big biceps and a treasured chest.

This chapter shows you how you use your arm and chest muscles on a daily basis — and how to exercise them. Before you start your exercise program, I recommend that you do the Home Fitness Evaluation in Chapter 8. This evaluation helps you determine your current fitness level (deconditioned or conditioned) so that you can create a workout program that works for you. You can find all the exercises listed in this chapter on your personal *Exercise Program Chart* (Appendix A). Pick your favorite exercises and highlight them in your chart. Your recommended sets (the number of times you perform a series of exercises) and reps (the number of repetitions you perform in each set) are listed after each exercise in this chapter. Remember to warm up and then stretch your muscles before you begin to exercise (see Chapter 3), don't forget to breathe as you go and, of course, have fun.

Working Your Chest

Men usually strive to pump up their pecs (pectoral muscles in the chest). Take a walk through the gym someday and you'll probably find mostly men on the bench press machines. Many men place greater emphasis on doing chest exercises at the expense of other muscle groups. Women, on the other hand, tend to avoid increasing their chest muscles because they fear looking like a gladiator. Conversely, women may remember the saying, "We must, we must, we must increase our bust." So some women started pumping up their chests in hopes of increasing their breasts. I hate to disappoint you, but when a woman exercises her chest muscles, they never get huge (unless she takes steroids that happen to be an illegal and dangerous drug). Chest exercises don't increase breast size either, but these exercises do help keep breasts firm. This information doesn't mean you shouldn't work out your chest muscles if you're female. A muscularly balanced body is the key for everyone, so put an exercise program together that incorporates all of your major muscles. (See Figure 10-1 for an illustration of the chest muscles.)

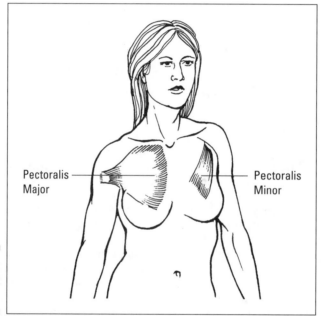

Pectoralis Major

Pectoralis Minor

Figure 10-1:
The chest
muscles.

Pectoral muscles (pecs) in both men and women make up the chest (shown in Figure 10-1). This muscle group helps you to push objects such as shopping carts, strollers, and furniture, and even to push some people if they get in your way at the sale rack. You sometimes take for granted how many jobs the pec muscles have. Without realizing it, you naturally use your pectoral muscles when you wash your car, garden, catch balls or other objects that come soaring at you, hug or squeeze your loved one or your dog, and even when you flush the toilet. Keeping your pec muscles strong not only helps you to look great, it can also make some of your daily tasks easier and help prevent injury while you play sports or do other activities. The following list shows you some of the exercises that you can do to work your chest:

✔ Push-ups

✔ Flys

✔ Straight-arm pullovers

Push-ups

When you think of push-ups, you probably imagine Marines at drill camp, but doing push-ups on your knees is a less difficult way to exercise your arms. Make sure you perform your push-ups on a carpeted floor or exercise mat for greater comfort. Crossing your ankles won't make a difference in the difficulty of the exercise, but if you choose to do the traditional military style push-up and put your toes on the ground instead of your knees (the knee version is shown in Figure 10-2), you're definitely increasing the difficulty of the exercise. You can find an example of the military style of push-up in the muscle strength test in Chapter 8. In this exercise, it's important to exhale during the period of exertion. (That would be on your way up from the floor.)

TAMILEE SAYS

NO cheating on the bench press

During my years as an undergraduate student, I spent a lot of time in the gym training my muscles. At that time it really wasn't cool for women to lift weights, so the majority of my fellow weight lifters were men. I noticed how concerned these guys were with their pectoral muscles and how they tried to impress each other with the amount of weight they could bench press. So, being one of the only females around, I decided to make a statement and challenge their great strength. I asked some of the guys if they could lift the same amount of weight without using their legs, back, and other muscles to assist them when performing a bench press. In other words, I had them place their feet on the bench instead of the floor and bench press the same amount of weight. You see, these guys were able to lift more weight because they were, in a sense, cheating. Their legs and hips stabilized their backs and torsos during the lift so they could actually lift more weight. Guess what? They didn't come close to lifting the same amounts of weight. A true bench press is focused on working the pectoral muscles and incorporates the use of your shoulders and arms for assistance. When I asked these guys not to use their legs and backs for assistance, they had to decrease the total amount of weight they were lifting. Needless to say, I felt pretty cool at that moment.

1. **Start on the floor on your hands and knees; place your hands slightly wider than shoulder width apart.**

2. **Slowly lower your chest towards the floor and push yourself back up.**

   Keep your back straight and head in alignment with your spine.

Deconditioned Exerciser	Conditioned Exerciser
Sets = 1	Sets = 3
Reps = as many as you can	Reps = 10
Tips: Increase sets and reps after 6 weeks.	*Tips:* Increase reps to 12. Rest 1 minute between sets.
Caution: Don't arch your back and avoid locking your elbow joints. Keep your abs pulled in tightly.	

Figure 10-2: Try push-ups on your knees.

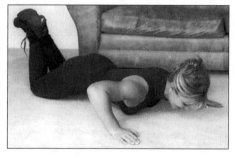 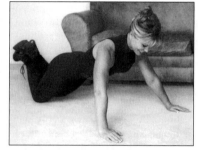

Flys

No, you aren't swatting flies or soaring through the sky with some imaginary wings for this exercise. The wings you're using for this move are your arms, and the only thing moving through the air are your hands holding on to a couple of dumbbells. As you can see in Figure 10-3, your arms move along an arc from above your chest to the sides of your chest. The best way to imagine this movement is to pretend you have a barrel lying on your chest and you must move your hands along the outside of it.

1. **Lie on your back with your back flat and feet firmly on the floor.**

2. **With the dumbbells in your hands, extend your arms toward the ceiling with your palms facing in.**

3. **Slowly lower your arms out to the sides and pull back into your starting position.**

   Keep the movement in your pecs and not in your arms.

Deconditioned Exerciser	Conditioned Exerciser
Sets = 1	Sets = 3
Reps = 8 to 10	Reps = 10 to 12
Weights = 3 to 5 lbs (1.4 to 2.3 kg)	Weights = 8 lbs or more (3.6 kg or more)
Tips: If you can't do 8 reps, do as many as you can. Increase sets and reps after 6 weeks.	*Tips:* Try this exercise on an incline bench.

Caution: Make sure your elbows are slightly bent and your wrists are straight. Your abs should be pulled in tightly to keep your back against the floor.

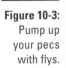

Figure 10-3: Pump up your pecs with flys.

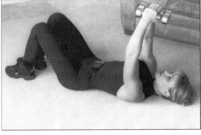 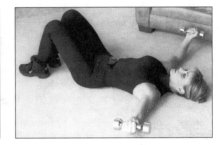

Straight-arm pullover

For the straight-arm pullover, make sure you hold the end of the dumbbell furthest from the floor, as shown in Figure 10-4. You can increase the benefit of this exercise as you lift the dumbbell by squeezing your pec muscles toward your sternum, the piece of bone between the top of your ribs. As you allow the dumbbell to lower to the floor, inhale. Exhale as you lift it over your head.

1. **Lie on your back with your feet firmly on the floor.**

2. **Hold one dumbbell in both hands and extend your arms overhead.**

3. **Slowly pull the dumbbell forward, stopping the movement over your chest.**

Deconditioned Exerciser	Conditioned Exerciser
Sets = 1	Sets = 3
Reps = 8 to 10	Reps = 10 to 12
Weights = 3 to 5 lbs (1.4 to 2.3 kg)	Weights = 8 lbs or more (3.6 kg or more)
Tips: Shorten your range of motion if you are having difficulty. Increase sets and reps after 6 weeks.	*Tips:* Try the pullover exercise on a straight bench and begin with the weight below the level of your head on the bench.

Caution: Be sure you aren't shrugging your shoulders as the weight passes back over your head. Keep your abdominals tight to support your back against the floor.

Figure 10-4: This move is more effective if you squeeze your pecs as you lift.

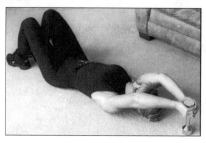 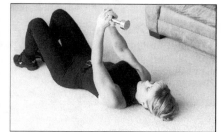

Working Your Arms

Strong arms are in. Some guys work their biceps just so they can flex their arms and recite that famous line, "This way to the beach." It is finally in fashion for women to have well-toned arm muscles, as well, and women are finding that summery sleeveless shirts are more flattering when their arms are firm. If you need a hint to determine if arm toning is necessary, just check to see if the lower half of your upper arm waves in the wind as you wave good-bye. If this is the case, you can wear long sleeves, but why not firm up your arms instead?

The muscles of your arm (shown in Figure 10-5), make it easy for you to bring things to or away from your body, like food, for example. What a thought . . . pushing food away? We could all probably lose a few pounds if we exercised such restraint when presented with the dessert tray.

The biceps (bis, guns, pipes) bend your arm forward and are used frequently, for everything from picking up children and pets to carrying grocery bags. The triceps (tris), which straighten your arm, oppose the biceps and are used to push things (or yourself) back and away. Strong biceps and triceps make the tasks in your daily life easier. The following exercises help you work your arms:

Biceps

✔ Hammer curl

✔ Wide curl

✔ Alternate curl

Triceps

✔ Overhead extension

✔ Kickbacks

✔ Triceps push-ups or dips

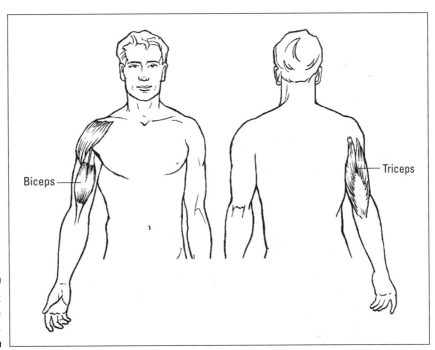

Figure 10-5:
The arm
muscles.

Forearm

| ✔ Two-wrist curl up
| ✔ Two-wrist curl down

Hammer curl

It's "Hammer Time" for your biceps. Add a dumbbell to firm, tone, and shape your arms. Just like a bicep curl, the range of motion that your hand moves through is from the side of your leg to the top of your shoulder, shown in Figure 10-6. You can emphasize the contraction to your bicep muscle by squeezing it as you lift the weight.

1. **Stand with your feet shoulder width apart and hold the dumbbells down by your sides.**

2. **Keeping your palms faced in toward your body, slowly curl your hands up to your shoulders.**

3. **Concentrate on squeezing your biceps at the top of the range of motion and then release your arms to their starting position.**

Deconditioned Exerciser	*Conditioned Exerciser*
Sets = 1	Sets = 3
Reps = 8 to 10	Reps = 10 to 12
Weights = 3 to 5 lbs. (1.4 to 2.3 kg)	Weights = 8 lbs. or more (3.6 kg or more)

Tips: Sit in a chair instead of standing. Increase sets and reps after 6 weeks.

Caution: Make sure your wrists are straight. Keep your abdominals tightened to support your back. Don't swing your arms through the range of motion; stay in control of the weight and your movement.

Wide curl

The wide curl is like doing a bicep curl in a "W" pattern (see Figure 10-7). By raising the dumbbells so that they end up outside of your shoulders, not in front of you, you can contract your bicep muscle slightly further than the traditional bicep curl does.

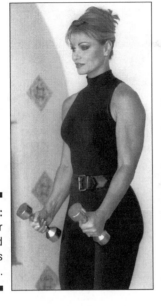 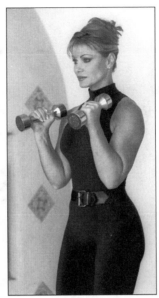

Figure 10-6:
No hammer
is required
for this
exercise.

1. **Stand with your feet shoulder width apart and hold the dumbbells next to your sides.**

2. **With your palms facing forward and hands slightly angled outward, curl your hands toward your shoulders.**

3. **Squeeze your biceps at the top of the motion and slowly release your arms to their starting position.**

Deconditioned Exerciser	*Conditioned Exerciser*
Sets = 1	Sets = 3
Reps = 8 to 10	Reps = 10 to 12
Weights = 3 to 5 lbs (1.4 to 2.3 kg)	Weights = 8 lbs or more (3.6 kg or more)

Tips: Begin with a light weight; this angle is more difficult than others. Increase sets and reps after 6 weeks.

Caution: Keep your wrists straight throughout the range of motion and keep your arms facing away from the body. Squeeze at the top of the range of motion. Be careful not to arch your back to help out with the lifting.

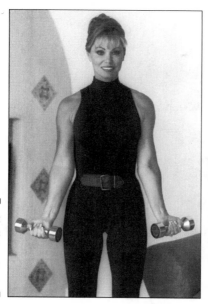 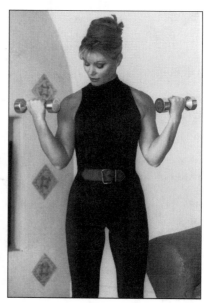

Figure 10-7:
Your arms
form a "W"
for the
wide curl.

Alternate curl

This is an exercise where one bicep gets to rest while you give the other your total concentration. Think about increasing the weight you're lifting because you're only lifting one hand at a time and have more energy to do each repetition (as shown in Figure 10-8).

1. **Stand with your feet shoulder width apart.**

2. **Hold the dumbbells by your sides with your palms facing away from your body.**

3. **Slowly lift one hand toward your shoulder, squeezing your biceps at the top.**

4. **Release your arm back to its starting position and repeat the exercise using your other arm.**

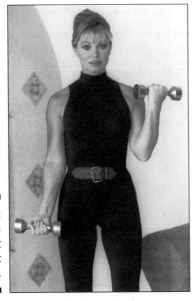 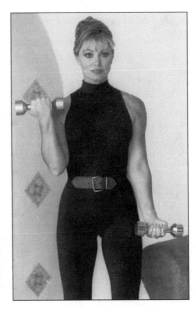

Figure 10-8:
Alternate
curls: take it
one arm at
a time.

Deconditioned Exerciser	Conditioned Exerciser
Sets = 1	Sets = 3
Reps = 8 to 10	Reps = 10 to 12
Weights = 3 to 5 lbs (1.4 to 2.3 kg)	Weights = 8 lbs or more (3.6 kg or more)
Tips: Try a seated position to support your back. Increase sets and reps after 6 weeks.	*Tips:* Begin with 5 lbs if 8 lbs is too heavy.

Caution: Be sure your wrists are straight and the rotation is coming from your forearm. Keep your abdominals tightened to support your back. Don't use your body's momentum to lift the weight, and don't rock your torso back and forth to lift the weights.

Overhead extension

If you're having difficulty maintaining proper body posture for this exercise, (like keeping your feet shoulder width apart and not arching your back extensively), try sitting in a chair. A chair helps you keep your back from swaying out and focuses your attention on the muscles in the back of your upper arms (triceps). Figure 10-9 shows the standing version.

1. **Stand with your feet together and knees slightly bent.**

2. **Hold one or both dumbbells (depending on the weight recommendations listed below) in both hands over your head.**

3. **Keeping your elbows close to your head, slowly lower the weight behind you.**

4. **Take the weight back to your starting position by extending your elbows and squeezing your triceps.**

Deconditioned Exerciser	Conditioned Exerciser
Sets = 1	Sets = 3
Reps = 8 to 10	Reps = 10 to 12
Weights = 3 to 5 lbs (1.4 to 2.3 kg)	Weights = 8 lbs or more (3.6 kg or more)
Tips: Try the exercise seated if you find it difficult. Increase sets and reps after 6 weeks.	*Tips:* Increase weight if this exercise becomes too easy.

Caution: Keep your abs tightened so that you don't arch your back. Make sure your elbows don't flare too far away from your head — that's cheating. Above all, don't smack yourself in the head with your weights.

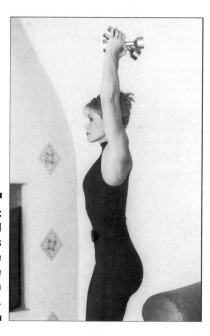 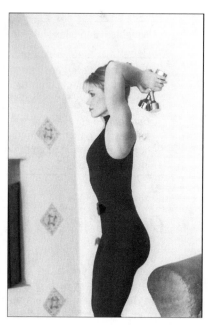

Figure 10-9: Overhead extensions can also be done while you sit in a chair.

Kickbacks

Although you may want to kick back and relax on the couch, I prefer that you kick back some weight and improve the strength of your tricep muscles, as Figure 10-10 shows. It's important to be cautious about your back in this exercise. If you tend to have back problems, you may prefer to sit in a chair and lean forward (chest toward your knees) to do your kickbacks.

1. **Stand with your feet together and hold the dumbbells by your side.**

2. **Bend from the waist so that your back is flat with a slight arch in it.**

3. **Bring your elbows up so that the dumbbells are next to your side and your palms are facing the sides of your legs.**

4. **Slowly extend your elbows, pushing the weight behind you.**

5. **As you push the weight back, rotate your palms to the ceiling. As you return the weight to the starting position, rotate your palms back to the sides of your legs.**

6. **Squeeze your triceps at the top of the range of motion (the point where your elbows are fully extended) and release them to their starting position.**

Deconditioned Exerciser	Conditioned Exerciser
Sets = 1	Sets = 3
Reps = 8 to 10	Reps = 10 to 12
Weights = 3 to 5 lbs (1.4 to 2.3 kg)	Weights = 8 lbs or more (3.6 kg or more)
Tips: Try sitting in a chair for support. Increase sets and reps after 6 weeks. Start off by working one arm at a time and alternate.	*Tips:* Extend both arms at the same time for an advanced option.

Caution: Keep your back straight and your head in alignment with your spine. Don't forget to keep your abdominals tight to support your back. Your elbows need to stay right next to your side so that the movement is concentrated in your triceps.

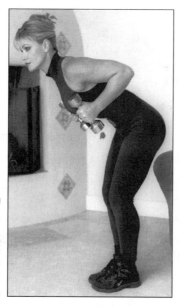 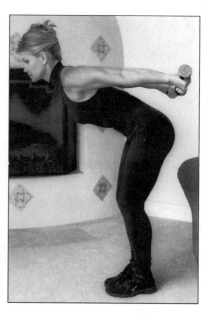

Figure 10-10:
Kickbacks . . .
and I don't
mean
relaxing!

Tricep push-ups or dips

Figure 10-11 shows one of my favorite arm exercises, because I like it and can do it anywhere. You don't need equipment — just your own body weight. It may look like an uncomfortable exercise, but if you follow my hints, you'll see the benefits this old-time exercise can offer you. Place your hands in a comfortable position slightly off the edge of the platform that you're using. Don't place them in an extremely flexed position and then put extra pressure on them as you're dipping your body weight up and down. Your wrists can become uncomfortable if they are hyper-extended, which means your wrists are flexed to about 90 degrees, and the tops of your hands are bent towards your forearm.

1. **Place your hands on the edge of a chair and bring your hips off the edge. Keep your feet on the floor and either bend your knees to make it easier, or straighten your legs out in front of you to make the exercise more difficult.**

2. **Slowly lower your body weight down until your elbows are bent to a 90-degree angle, and then push yourself back up to your starting position.**

3. **Squeeze your triceps at the top of the range of motion (the point where your elbows are fully extended).**

Deconditioned Exerciser	Conditioned Exerciser
Sets = 1	Sets = 3
Reps = as many as you can	Reps = 10 to 12
Tips: Bend your legs at a 90-degree angle to make it easier. Limit your range of motion and don't go down too far (only bend your elbow to about a 45-degree angle instead of 90 degrees). Increase sets and reps after 6 weeks.	*Tips:* Extend legs straight to increase difficulty. For even greater difficulty, place your legs on a chair and dip your body down between the two chairs.

Caution: Keep your elbows parallel to each other; be careful that your elbows don't bend less than a 90-degree angle. Don't hyperextend your wrists; keep them straight. Move your body through a full range of motion; your elbows should fully flex so that your body dips to the lowest point, and then you should extend your elbows and bring yourself all the way back up. Basically, I mean no short little dips.

Figure 10-11: Make sure the furniture you use for this exercise is stable.

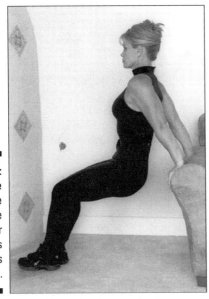
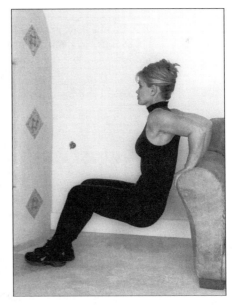

Two-wrist curl-up

Flexing your wrists may sound like a meaningless exercise, but many people who play sports like golf and tennis swear that the exercise shown in Figure 10-12 (and the next) enhances their abilities. The curl-up focuses on wrist flexion. When your fingers are aligned with your forearm, your wrists are straight. If I ask you to make a fist by curling your fingers toward your forearm, you are flexing your wrist. Now do it with a dumbbell to increase your strength.

1. **Stand with your feet together and hold the dumbbells against the front of your thighs.**

2. **With your palms up, carefully flex from your wrists, pulling your hands up.**

3. **Extend your hands back down to the thighs.**

Deconditioned Exerciser	*Conditioned Exerciser*
Sets = 1	Sets = 3
Reps = 5 to 8	Reps = 8 to 10
Weights = 1 to 3 lbs (0.5 to 1.4 kg)	Weights = 5 lbs or more (2.3 kg or more)
Tips: Do one hand at a time. Try the exercise in a seated position. Increase sets and reps after 6 weeks.	*Tips:* Hold the contraction for 2 seconds.

Caution: Move slowly and control your motion as you flex your wrists. Don't allow the weight to drop down.

Two-wrist curl-down

The exercise in Figure 10-13 requires wrist extension. When your flex your wrist you bring your fingers toward your body, so if you extend it, you're moving them away from your body. While doing the curl-down, the tops of your hands move backward toward the tops of your forearms.

1. **Stand with your feet together and hold the dumbbells against the front of your thighs.**

2. **With your palms facing your legs, pull your hands upward from the wrists and then release them back down.**

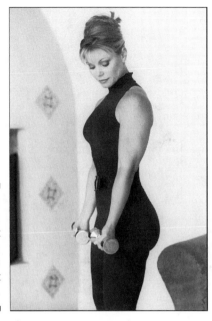 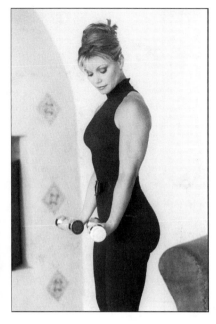

Figure 10-12:
The
two-wrist
curl-up
requires
light
weights.

Deconditioned Exerciser	*Conditioned Exerciser*
Sets = 1	Sets = 3
Reps = 5 to 8	Reps = 8 to 10
Weights = 1 to 3 lbs (0.5 to 1.4 kg)	Weights = 5 lbs or more (2.3 kg or more)
Tips: Try the exercise seated. Increase sets and reps after 6 weeks.	*Tips:* Hold the contraction for 2 seconds.

Caution: Be sure the movement stays only in the wrists, not in the arms and shoulders. Keep your knees slightly bent and abs in.

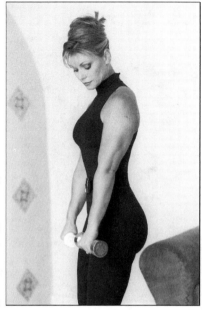 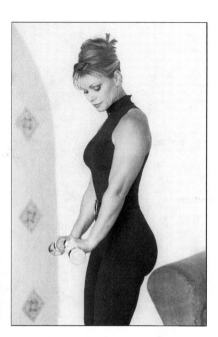

Figure 10-13:
The two-wrist curl-down strengthens your forearms.

Chapter 11

Carry the Weight of the World: Back and Shoulder Exercises

*I*n Greek mythology, the Titan Atlas was condemned to carry the weight of the world on his shoulders. Fortunately, he had the shoulder and back muscles to do it. Sometimes the stress you carry can be just as heavy as the weight of the globe that burdened Atlas. By strengthening the muscles of your back and shoulders, you can carry out daily activities with greater ease and lower your risk of injury. Warming up and stretching (see Chapter 3) are an important part of your exercise routine and can help you eliminate some of the stress you tend to carry in these specific muscle groups.

This chapter shows you how you use, and how to exercise, your back and shoulder muscles, and you can find the exercises from this chapter listed in your personal *Exercise Program Chart* (Appendix A). It's a good idea to do the Home Fitness Evaluation (in Chapter 8) before you design your workout program. This evaluation helps you determine your current fitness level (deconditioned or conditioned) so that you can create a workout that works for you.

Your fitness level determines how many sets and reps I recommend you do. (Reps is short for repetitions, and those are the number of times you should lift a particular weight. Sets are the number of times you should repeat the repetitions.) It's important to follow this simple rule when you exercise: *Ex*hale as you *ex*ert energy, which means during the most difficult part of the exercise. Inhale on the opposite direction. For example, if I ask you to do an overhead press (see Figure 11-10), you would exhale as you push the weight over your head and inhale as you return it to your side. After you choose your favorite exercises or make up your own, highlight them in the *Exercise Program Chart* (Appendix A)

Back to Work

What's your answer if I ask you, "Which are stronger: your abdominal or your lower back muscles?"

Bet you answered the abdominals. Most people do, especially considering how focused many people are on strengthening their abdominals. Actually, your back muscles tend to be stronger — and they need to be, because they are at work all day long. However, even though your back generally consists of strong muscle groups, many people injure their backs frequently due to overuse, lower back weakness, and incorrect exercising techniques. The best way to decrease your risk of back injury and pain is to properly exercise all of your back muscles. Don't neglect a few to benefit the others. In addition, by strengthening your supporting muscles like the abdominals and the legs, you can avoid relying solely on your back muscles for everyday activities.

Your back muscles are made up of four major muscle groups, the latissimus dorsi, trapezius, rhomboids, and the erector spinae, shown in Figure 11-1.

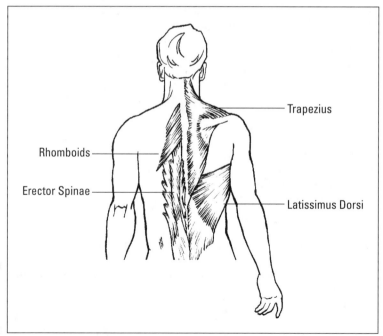

Figure 11-1:
Back
muscles.

The *latissimus dorsi* (lats, wings) is one of the largest muscle groups in your body and the largest in your back. The main function of this muscle group is to assist your arms in pulling things toward your body, like the leash attached to your runaway dog, or to pull yourself upward, like on a chin-up bar.

Your *trapezius* muscles (traps) aid you in shrugging your shoulders, as if you're saying "So what?" or "I don't know." You may notice that your upper trapezius muscle tends to get tight if you are feeling stressed out. Many people tense their shoulders up to their necks when dealing with stress. The tightening of these upper trapezius muscles causes even greater tension. When dealing with stressful situations, give yourself a relaxation break and a stretch (see the section on stress-busting stretches in Chapter 18).

Did your mother ever tell you to pull your shoulders back and stand up straight? If you have heard this before and obeyed, you contracted your *rhomboid* muscles. These muscles, when contracted, pull your shoulder blades together and help you maintain good posture.

One of the most important muscle groups in our body is in our back. This muscle group is the *erector spinae* (lower back), and its main function is to erect your spine. In addition to extending your spine upright, this muscle group also supports your torso in everything you do. For example, when you bend over to pick up a child, you use your abdominals in order to flex your torso forward. As you stand up, you use your erector spinae to extend and straighten your torso to an upright position. The best way to avoid unnecessary back injury is to use your legs and buns to stand up, especially when you're lifting something heavy. When doing the exercises I list for the erector spinae, you're focusing on strengthening the area of your lower back. If you currently have a lower-back injury or are prone to lower-back pain, please consult your physician or physical therapist for a list of exercises that can benefit you the most.

The following exercises can help you work your back.

- Shoulder raises
- One-arm row
- Kneeling two-arm row
- Superman
- Alternate leg lift

"I Don't Know" shoulder raises

I'm sure at times you shrug your shoulders when asked a question you don't know the answer to. You may even be practicing it each time your boss asks you when your report will be done. Now that you've got the motion down, just add a little weight to it. Grab your dumbbells or a barbell and hold them in front of your thighs with your palms facing down, as shown in Figure 11-2. Now just repeatedly say, "I don't know."

1. **Stand with your feet hip-width apart and hold the dumbbells in front of your thighs, palms facing down.**

2. **Shrug your shoulders toward your ears and then relax them.**

Deconditioned Exerciser	Conditioned Exerciser
Sets = 1	Sets = 3
Reps = 8 to 10	Reps = 10 to 12
Weights = 1 to 2 lb (0.5 to .9 kg)	Weights = 5 to 10 lb (2.3 to 4.5 kg)
Tips: Sit in a chair to begin. Increase sets and reps after 6 weeks.	*Tips:* Hold the lift for 2 seconds and release.

Caution: Keep your knees slightly bent, and tighten your abdominals for torso support. Be careful not to roll your shoulders. Think about raising your shoulders straight up in a vertical motion.

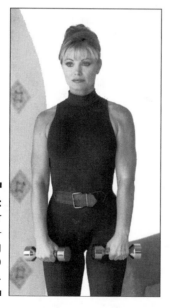
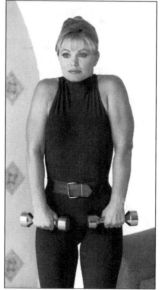

Figure 11-2:
Shoulder raise — shrugging your way to strength.

One-arm row (starting your mower)

It's easy to let your arm begin to swing through the movement in this exercise, but you have to pay attention to what you're doing. Think about drawing a line from your front foot diagonally up to your hip. The weight in your hand should begin at the beginning of your line, at your foot, and follow up to your hip. (Figure 11-3 shows you the movement.)

1. **Stand with your right foot about 12 inches (30.5 cm) in front of the left foot and hold a dumbbell in your left hand. Make sure your stance is stable and comfortable.**

2. **Bend forward, placing your right hand on your front (right) leg for support.**

3. **Extend your left hand down with your palm facing toward your body.**

4. **Slowly pull your elbow up while squeezing your shoulder blade and elbow in toward your spine.**

5. **Extend the arm back down and repeat on both sides.**

Deconditioned Exerciser	*Conditioned Exerciser*
Sets = 1	Sets = 3
Reps = 8 to 10 each side	Reps = 10 to 12 each side
Weights = 3 to 5 lb (1.4 to 2.3 kg)	Weights = 8 to 12 lb (3.6 to 5.4 kg)
Tips: Try sitting in a chair instead of standing. Increase sets and reps after 6 weeks.	
Caution: Be careful not to rotate your torso as you lift your elbow. Keep your torso straight. Don't excessively arch or round out your spine. Tighten your abdominals to help support your back, and keep your shoulders from shrugging up toward your ears.	

Kneeling two-arm row

The two-arm row shown in Figure 11-4 gives you a two-for-one deal as you exercise your back. This exercise may be more comfortable for you if you sit on the edge of a chair and lean your chest forward. In either position, concentrate on squeezing your shoulder blades together and contracting the muscles of your upper back.

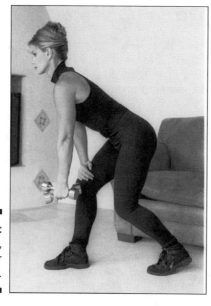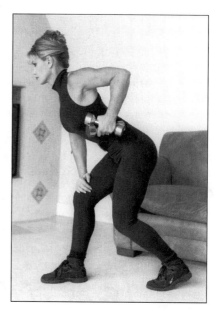

Figure 11-3:
Row, row,
row, your
arms.

1. **Lower yourself down on one knee and lean your torso against your front leg.**

2. **Place the weights in your hands and extend your arms to the floor with your palms facing in.**

3. **Slowly pull your elbows back and inward as your hands separate.**

4. **Release your arms to their starting position.**

Deconditioned Exerciser	*Conditioned Exerciser*
Sets = 1	Sets = 3
Reps = 8 to 10	Reps = 10 to 12
Weights = 3 to 5 lbs (1.4 to 2.3 kg)	Weights = 8 to 10 lbs (3.6 to 5.4 kg)
Tips: Sit in a chair and lean forward instead of kneeling. Increase sets and reps after 6 weeks.	

Caution: Keep your shoulder blades pulled down toward your waist. Avoid allowing the muscles of your torso to assist you by lifting your chest away from your front knee. Tighten your abdominals to support your back.

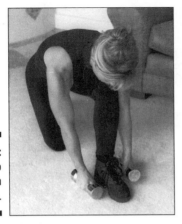
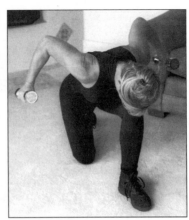

Figure 11-4:
Rowing to
the finish
line.

Superman

Atlas may be strong, but Superman can fly, and this exercise may be how he developed such great flying form. Whether you get from one place to another by flying or walking, your back muscles need to be strong. This exercise, shown in Figure 11-5, may look simple, but it's effective for developing strength in your back.

1. **Lie on the floor with your arms and legs extended in a linear position.**

2. **Lift one arm and the opposite leg, simultaneously, away from the floor.**

3. **Release and repeat using your other leg and arm.**

Deconditioned Exerciser	*Conditioned Exerciser*
Sets = 1	Sets = 3
Reps = 8 to 10 each side	Reps = 10 to 12 each side

Tips: You can add 1 to 2 lb (0.5 to 0.9 kg) hand weights to increase resistance. Think about reaching out as if someone is pulling your leg and arm.

Caution: Keep your head in alignment with your spine. (Don't look up to check yourself out in the mirror.) Move slowly, controlling your movements. Tighten your abdominals and don't arch your back.

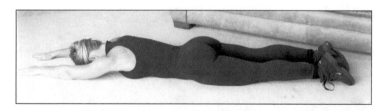

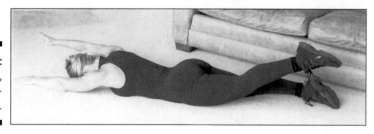

Figure 11-5:
Superman,
or Super-
woman.

Alternate leg lift

This exercise, shown in Figure 11-6, is a level up in difficulty from the Superman (described in the preceding section). You have to control any swaying in your stomach by tightening your abdominals.

1. **Place your hands and knees on the floor and keep your back straight and your neck aligned with your spine.**

2. **Lift one leg up, straightening the knee, and then release it back down to its starting position.**

3. **Repeat and switch to your other leg.**

Deconditioned Exerciser	Conditioned Exerciser
Sets = 1	Sets = 3
Reps = 8 to 10 each side	Reps = 10 to 12 each side

Tips: Make sure you are comfortable doing the Superman exercise earlier in this chapter before you try this one.

Caution: When lifting your leg, be sure your motion is controlled. Don't swing your leg up and down, which allows your stomach to sway and causes an excessive arch in your back. Tighten your abdominals to support your back.

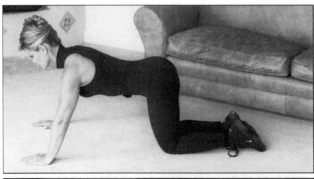

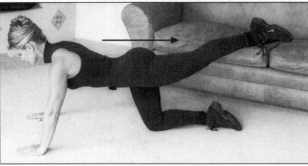

Figure 11-6:
Avoid an
extensive
arch in your
back for
this
exercise.

Working Your Shoulders

In the late 1980s and early 1990s, fashion designers decided to help women pump up their shoulders by placing shoulder pads in clothing. These superficial shoulders were a wonderful idea because the bigger your shoulders are the smaller your waist and hips look. But what happens when you're on the beach in a bathing suit? Here come your hips for all the world to see. As time went by, women learned that if they exercise their shoulders like many men do, they can actually create strong, well-defined shoulders that keep their waists and hips looking narrow no matter what they wear. Men learned this trick long ago. Men's suits are designed with shoulder pads to create the look of strong, broad shoulders, but when the time comes to put on casual wear, it rarely comes with muscle-enhancing devices. Members of both genders have found that if they want strong, defined shoulders, they must work on creating the real thing!

The shoulder muscles (shown in Figure 11-7) consist of the *deltoids*, or delts, (anterior, medial, and posterior) and the *rotator cuff* muscles (rotators). The muscles that make up your deltoids cover and protect the shoulder joint and allow you to move your arms up, down, to the side, and behind you. Having strong deltoids not only helps the look of your overall figure, regardless of your gender, but also helps you lift things and throw a good pitch.

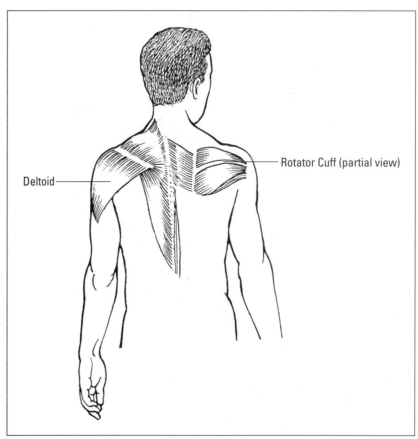

Deltoid

Rotator Cuff (partial view)

Figure 11-7:
Shoulder
muscles.

The rotator cuff muscles do just what their name implies: They rotate your arm in and out and protect the cuff of your shoulder joint. Athletes like baseball players and golfers frequently injure these muscles. Injury of the rotator cuff is often caused by the repeated swinging motion such athletes perform with their arms. Whether or not you are involved in these sports, it's important to work these muscles. You don't see any major physical change by exercising your rotator cuffs, so you may have a tendency to overlook them. You don't want to wait, however, until you have a shoulder injury to realize the value of strengthening the rotator cuff muscles. Injury to the rotator cuff muscles is so common, in fact, that in a study of people who died at age 70, 75 percent of them had unrepaired rotator cuff injuries.

Work your shoulders with the following exercises.

Deltoids

✔ Side raises

✔ Rear delt lifts

✔ Overhead press

Rotator Cuff

✔ External rotation

✔ Internal rotation

Side raises (flap your wings)

Figure 11-8 shows you that this exercise is similar to making angels in the snow, except that you don't lift your arms any higher than your shoulders. Think of it as having your wings clipped.

1. **Stand with your feet hip-width apart and hold the dumbbells next to the sides of your legs, palms facing in.**

2. **Slowly lift your arms out to your sides and away from your body, and then release them. Don't lift the weights higher than your shoulder level.**

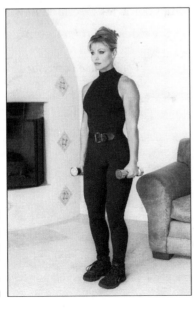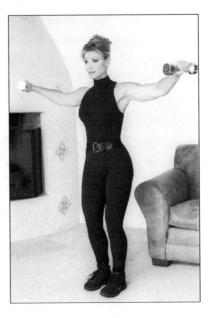

Figure 11-8:
Side raises:
Ready for
take-off.

Deconditioned Exerciser	Conditioned Exerciser
Sets = 1	Sets = 3
Reps = 8 to 10	Reps = 10 to 12
Weights = 3 to 5 lbs (1.4 to 2.3 kg)	Weights = 8 to 10 lbs (3.6 to 4.5 kg)
Tips: Begin the exercise seated to help support your back. Or stagger your for more back support. Increase sets and reps after 6 weeks.	*Tips:* Lift the weights up in 3 seconds and resist down in 1 second. (In other words, don't let the weight fall quickly.
Caution: Do not lift the weights higher than your shoulder level. Maintain straight wrists and keep your palms facing the floor as you reach the top of your motion. Keep your knees slightly bent and tighten your abdominals.	

Rear delt lift

Bringing up the rear can help develop your posterior (rear) deltoid muscles. As you can see in Figure 11-9, the weight is held in front of you at the starting position, then pulled up toward your back for a full contraction of the muscle.

1. **Stand with one foot in front of the other and bend slightly forward from your waist, keeping your back straight.**

2. **Place your palms together with your arms extended downward.**

3. **Slowly raise your arms out to the sides and then lower them.**

Deconditioned Exerciser	Conditioned Exerciser
Sets = 1	Sets = 3
Reps = 8 to 10	Reps = 10 to 12
Weights = 3 to 5 lbs (1.4 to 2.3 kg)	Weights = 8 to 10 lbs (3.6 to 4.5 kg)
Tips: Try the exercise in a seated position. Increase sets and reps after 6 weeks.	
Caution: Tighten your abdominals for support. Keep both knees slightly bent, and keep your torso straight during the execution of the movement.	

Overhead press

Think of this exercise as lifting the world off your shoulders and up into the sky. As you perform the exercise shown in Figure 11-10, start with the dumbbells just above your shoulders and aligned next to your ears.

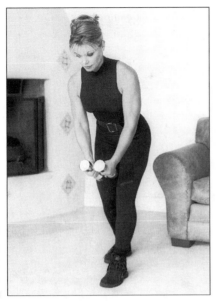 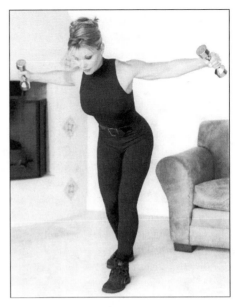

Figure 11-9:
Bringing up
the rear.

1. **Stand with your feet hip-width apart.**

2. **Hold the dumbbells at your shoulders and next to your ears with your palms facing forward.**

3. **Slowly extend the weight overhead as you straighten your arms, and then release your arms back down to shoulder level.**

Deconditioned Exerciser	Conditioned Exerciser
Sets = 1	Sets = 3
Reps = 8 to 10	Reps = 10 to 12
Weights = 3 to 5 lbs (1.4 to 2.3 kg)	Weights = 8 to 10 lbs (3.6 to 4.5 kg)

Tips: Sit on a chair with your feet flat on the floor. Stagger your feet to support your back. Alternate your arms instead of lifting both simultaneously. Increase sets and reps after 6 weeks.

Caution: Keep your back straight, with no excessive arching, and keep your knees slightly bent. Make sure the weight is in line with your ears and not in front of your face. If you have any shoulder pain when performing this exercise, you may have a rotator cuff injury. If this is the case, get checked out by a physician or a therapist before continuing this exercise.

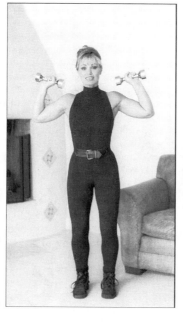 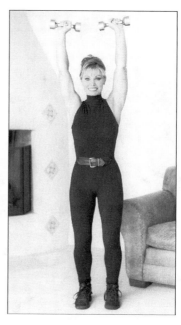

Figure 11-10:
Take the
weight of
the world
off your
shoulders.

External rotation

Have you ever served food? Compare the exercise in Figure 11-11 to holding a tray in front of you (with your palms facing up), and then moving it out and away from your body, which means you are externally rotating at your shoulder joint.

1. **Stand with your feet hip-width apart.**

2. **Bring your elbows into your waist and keep them bent at a 90-degree angle.**

3. **With your palms facing the ceiling, slowly rotate your arms out to the sides of your body, squeezing your shoulder blades together. Return your arms to their starting position.**

Deconditioned Exerciser	*Conditioned Exerciser*
Sets = 1	Sets = 3
Reps = 8 to 10	Reps = 10 to 12
Weights = 0 to 2 lbs (0 to 0.9 kg)	Weights = 3 to 5 lbs (1.4 to 2.3 kg)
Tips: Make your movements slow and controlled, holding for a moment on your outward contraction. Increase sets and reps after 6 weeks.	
Caution: Keep your wrists straight. Keep your elbows in close to your body.	

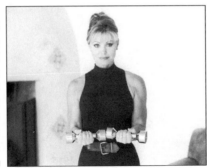 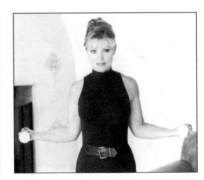

Figure 11-11: External rotation (which may help you the next time you serve food!).

Internal rotation

This exercise works your rotator cuff muscles using internal rotation at your shoulder joint. Your hands should be next to your head when you begin this exercise (as shown in Figure 11-12) and end up alongside your waist.

1. **Stand with your feet hip-width apart.**

2. **Bring both arms to a box position (elbows up at shoulder level and hands next to your head with your palms facing away from your body).**

3. **Keep your elbows still and rotate your shoulders so that your forearms move from the sides of your head down to the sides of your body. Your palms will now be facing behind you.**

4. **Return to the starting position and repeat.**

Deconditioned Exerciser	*Conditioned Exerciser*
Sets = 1	Sets = 3
Reps = 8 to 10	Reps = 10 to 12
Weights = 0 to 2 lbs (0 to 0.9 kg)	Weights = 3 to 5 lbs (1.4 to 2.3 kg)
Tips: Make all movements slow and controlled. Increase sets and reps after 6 weeks.	
Caution: Be sure to keep your elbows aligned with your shoulders. Keep your knees slightly bent.	

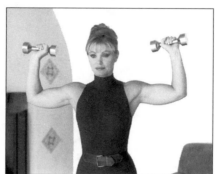 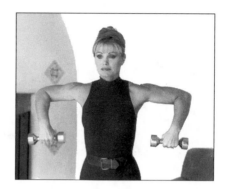

Figure 11-12:
Internal
rotation
works your
rotator cuff
muscles.

Part IV
Lower-Body Workouts

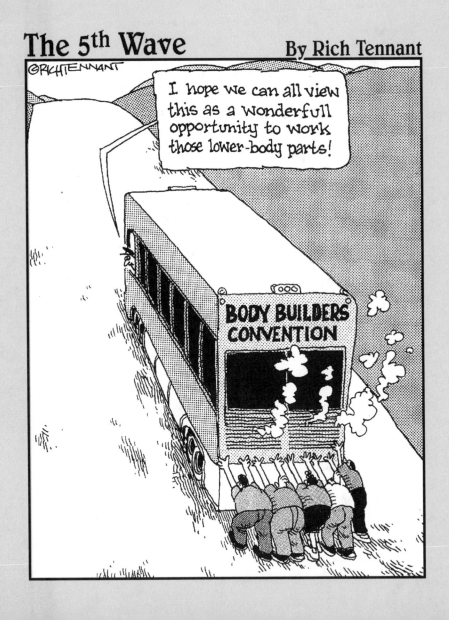

The 5th Wave   By Rich Tennant

I hope we can all view this as a wonderfull opportunity to work those lower-body parts!

BODY BUILDERS CONVENTION

In this part . . .

1 move the emphasis on down to your buns, legs, and thighs in this part. If you're looking to tone and tighten your lower body, you can find several exercises to shape up these muscles. You can also find plenty of information on how to keep your lower body in shape, and I give you my personal favorite bun strengtheners (like squats and lunges) as well as a few stories about how I stay fit.

Chapter 12

Crunch Time: Awesome Abdominal Exercises

- -

In This Chapter

▶ Recognizing different abdominal muscles and their functions

▶ Exercising your abdominal muscles

▶ Using the correct form for abdominal workouts

- -

Absolutely abs! Exercises for the abdominal muscles are in demand from men and women alike. Some people desire to develop a six pack while others just want to keep their bellies from rolling over their belts. It doesn't matter which point you are at in toning up your abdominal muscles (or abs, for short); this chapter shows you what they can do for you and how to exercise them. Before you get started, check out Chapter 8 to determine your current fitness level (deconditioned or conditioned). This is the Home Fitness Evaluation. One part of this evaluation is to test your muscular endurance, which is done by counting how many sit-ups you can do in the time allotted. After you've assessed your level, you can design the workout program that works best for you. From there, look in Appendix A at your personal *Exercise Program Chart* to find the exercises you have chosen from this and other chapters. You can also list how many repetitions (reps) you plan on doing for each exercise. You're ready to start crunching those abs once you've warmed up and stretched your muscles (see Chapter 3).

As a final note, I would like to remind you that holding your breath while exercising your abs will not make the exercise any easier. I have seen people's faces turn beet-red from holding their breath. It's a good thing they were all lying down or they would have passed out. The key to breathing while doing your ab work is to exhale as you contract your ab muscles and inhale as you release the contraction. Try it. You may find you can do more sit-ups than you thought.

Crunching Those Abs

Your abdominal muscles consist of four muscle groups: the rectus abdominis, external and internal obliques, and the transverse abdominis. (Besides the common term abs, good nicknames for the abdominals are *six pack* and *washboard;* however, you don't want anyone to say *spare tire* or *love handles* when referring to your physique!) The abdominal muscles (shown in Figure 12-1) work as a team to help support your lower back and create torso stability. The abs enable you to bend forward, bend backward, and rotate the trunk of your body.

The longest of the four muscles is the *rectus abdominis,* which spans from your sternum (the lowest point of the chest bone) to your pelvic bone, and helps you to curl your torso forward — like you do in an abdominal crunch. The *external* and *internal obliques* run diagonally up and down the sides of the mid portion of your torso. Having good obliques and a little rhythm can get you a spot as a finalist in the next twist and shout contest. The *transverse abdominis* is the muscle that contracts when you cough or sneeze. This is the muscle you tighten up or suck in when you're at the beach or trying to fit into the outfit you bought five years ago.

The following exercises allow you to work your abdominals.

- ✔ Lower 90-degree contraction
- ✔ Curl-up
- ✔ Crunch
- ✔ Crossover
- ✔ Side lateral slide

Tighten your abs!

"Tighten your abs" is a common tip listed in almost every exercise. For example, when doing a bicep curl, you can contract your abs as you contract your bicep muscle. By tightening or contracting your abdominal muscles as you perform an exercise, you help support your back and stabilize the trunk of your body. Your ab muscles also receive the added bonus of additional workout time because you are exerting them (contracting and releasing) during the majority of your exercises.

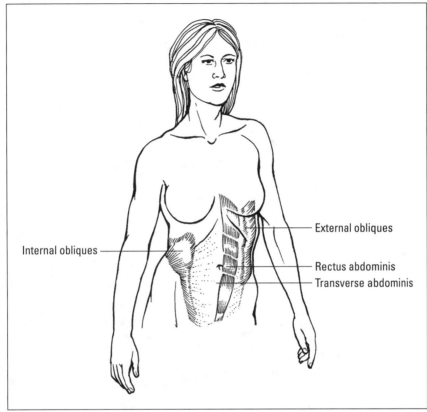

Figure 12-1:
The muscles everyone wants to work: abdominals.

Internal obliques

External obliques

Rectus abdominis

Transverse abdominis

Lower 90-degree contraction (or hip lift)

It's easy to relax and want to just close your eyes in this position, but keep focused and concentrate on your exercise. As you can see in Figure 12-2, the movement of your legs from starting position to the ending point is short. Looks may be deceiving, because this exercise requires that you concentrate on tightening the lower portion of your abdominal muscles in order to lift your hips off the ground and bring your knees up in the direction of your chest.

1. **Lie on your back with your knees and hips bent at a 90-degree angle (resting your feet on a couch or chair) and place your hands behind your head.**

2. **Slowly lift your feet off the couch and pull your knees in toward your chest. Keep your head relaxed on the floor.**

3. **As you release, bringing your feet back to the couch, keep your lower back on the floor.**

Inhale as you lower your feet and exhale as you pull your knees back in.

Deconditioned Exerciser	*Conditioned Exerciser*
Sets = 1	Sets = 3
Reps = as many as you can	Reps = 25
Tips: Increase sets and reps after 6 weeks.	*Tips:* Do the same movement without resting your feet on a couch. Add a dumbbell between your legs to increase the resistance to your abs.

Caution: Don't use your legs to kick or swing through the movement. Focus on bringing your hips and pelvis up to your ribcage.

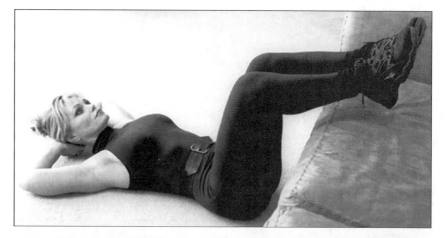

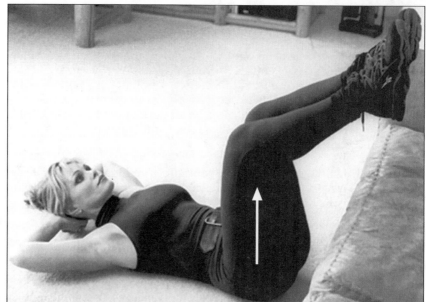

Figure 12-2:
Lower
90-degree
contraction.

Curl it up

The goal of this exercise is not to see how high you can curl your torso up, but to lift your shoulders off the ground high enough to feel your abdominals become tight. Figure 12-3 demonstrates this traditional, yet effective exercise.

1. **Lie on your back, rest your feet on a couch or chair, and place your hands behind your head.**

2. **Lift your head and shoulders off the floor as you lift your torso up toward the ceiling and in toward your hips.**

3. **Release your torso back to the floor in a slow, controlled motion.**

    Exhale as you contract up and inhale as you resist down.

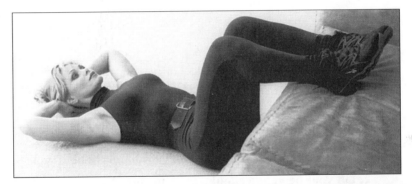

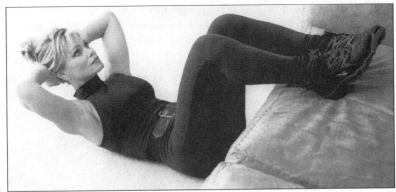

Figure 12-3:
The straight forward curl-up.

Deconditioned Exerciser	*Conditioned Exerciser*
Sets = 1	Sets = 3
Reps = 10 or more	Reps = 25
Tips: Lift your shoulders toward the ceiling. Increase sets and reps after 6 weeks.	*Tips:* Change your count to 3 seconds as you lift up and 1 second to resist down. Place a dumbbell in your hands behind your head as you lift your chest up.

Caution: Keep your head and neck in alignment with your spine (don't do a "neck up"). Keep your chin off your chest by pretending you have an orange between your chin and your chest. Maintain the strength of your abs throughout the movement to help protect any back injury. Finally, keep your elbows out rather than pointed toward the ceiling.

Crunch it up

Don't get into a crunch for time; get into a crunch to work your abs! This exercise (shown in Figure 12-4) puts together the first two in this chapter. An ab crunch requires you to lift your hips and chest simultaneously to get an intense ab exercise. Yes, that means it will be more difficult.

1. **Lie on your back with your knees bent at a 90-degree angle, feet resting on a couch or chair and your hands behind your head.**

2. **Lift your head and shoulders up toward the ceiling (see "Curl it up," earlier in this chapter) and lift your knees in toward your chest simultaneously (see "Lower 90-degree contraction," also earlier in this chapter).**

3. **Keeping the mid and lower portion of your back on the floor, hold this tensed position for a moment and then release your pelvis and shoulders back to their starting positions.**

   Exhale as you contract your abs and lift your pelvis and shoulders off the ground. Inhale as you release them back down.

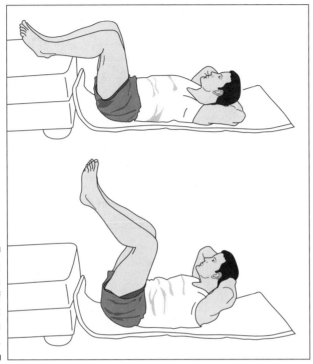

Figure 12-4:
Make the
most of
your abs:
Crunch
them.

Deconditioned Exerciser	Conditioned Exerciser
Sets = 1	Sets = 3
Reps = as many as you can	Reps = 25
Tips: Find a spot on the ceiling to focus on; this helps you maintain good alignment. Increase sets and reps after 6 weeks.	*Tips:* Change your count to crunch up in 1 second and lower down in 3 seconds. Place a dumbbell in your hands behind your head to increase the intensity.

Caution: Don't swing through the movement or allow momentum to take you through the motion. Keep your chin off your chest and keep your elbows out rather than pointed toward the ceiling.

Crossover for better obliques

It's time to cross over to the other side and give your obliques a chance to do their job, which is to rotate the trunk of your body from side to side. You may tend to pull on your head with your hands when you perform this exercise. This usually happens when you try to bring your elbow up to your knee as you crossover. If you look closely at Figure 12-5, you can notice that you're not required to bring your elbow to your knee. In fact, I would rather you think about directing your shoulder over toward your opposite knee. This strategy works your abs more and lessens the pull on your head.

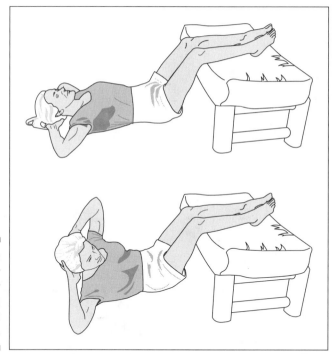

Figure 12-5:
Crossover
(or
squeezing
on an
angle).

1. **Lie on your back with your feet on the floor and knees bent, or rest your feet up on a couch at a 90-degree angle.**

2. **Place your hands behind your head with your elbows extended outward.**

3. **Slowly lift your left shoulder (NOT your elbow) to your right knee, crossing your body diagonally and contracting your oblique muscles.**

4. **Lower yourself to the starting position and repeat.**

5. **Repeat, using your right shoulder and crossing it to your left knee.**

   Exhale as you lift and cross shoulder; inhale as you lower back down.

Deconditioned Exerciser	*Conditioned Exerciser*
Sets = 1	Sets = 3
Reps = 10 or more each side	Reps = 20 each side
Tips: Rest your legs on a chair or couch to keep your back on the floor. Increase sets and reps after 6 weeks.	*Tips:* Increase difficulty by pulling your opposite knee in to meet your shoulder.

Caution: Maintain neutral alignment by keeping your chin off your chest. Don't twist your torso; just angle your shoulder toward your knee. Make sure your lower back doesn't arch up as you lower your shoulder. This arching can happen if you aren't resting your feet on a chair and your abs aren't strong.

Side lateral slide

As you can see, the movement in Figure 12-6 is not some kind of dance. It's just another exercise to tighten and tone your obliques. For some odd reason, I find this exercise more fun than the others. As long as you keep your head in line with your spine, all you have to do is slowly slide from side to side.

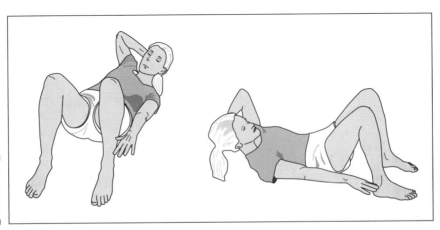

Figure 12-6: Side lateral slide.

1. Lie on your back with your knees bent and feet on the floor.

2. Place your right hand behind your head and lift your shoulders slightly off the floor.

3. With your left hand, reach or slide down the side of your body toward your left heel contracting your oblique muscles.

4. Repeat your reaches, exhaling as you reach down and inhaling as you return to the center position.

5. Switch hands and repeat on your other side.

Deconditioned Exerciser	Conditioned Exerciser
Sets =1	Sets = 3
Reps = 10 each side	Reps = 20 each side
Tips: Increase sets and reps after 6 weeks.	

Caution: Keep your chin off your chest and shoulders elevated slightly off the ground. Keep your lower back on the floor; no arching.

TIP

Make me laugh

Laughter gives your abdominals a workout. Have you ever said, "Stop making me laugh; my stomach hurts!"? Actually, your abs hurt because you're contracting them as you laugh. Try putting your hands on your abs next time you hear a good joke or go to a comedy show and you can feel your muscles contracting.

Sort of puts watching sitcoms in a whole new light, doesn't it? After all, if you're laughing at the show, you're exercising more than most couch potatoes. It's also a good idea to date someone who makes you laugh. Even if the date doesn't work out, at least you get a workout.

Chapter 13

Strong, Fit Legs: Leg Exercises

. . . .

In This Chapter

▶ Knowing (and loving) your leg muscles and their functions

▶ Exercising your legs

▶ Sidestepping mistakes and injuries while working your legs

. . . .

You don't have to be a runner to know the power of your legs. From infancy on, you learn that your legs are the body part that takes you where you want to go whether you choose to wobble, walk, skip, or run there.

This chapter shows you how you use your leg muscles and how to exercise them. Check out Chapter 8 and complete the Home Fitness Evaluation before starting your exercise program. This worksheet helps you determine your current fitness level (deconditioned or conditioned) so that you can create a workout that fits your needs. In that chapter, I've also included my suggestions on how many repetitions (*reps*) you should do of each exercise you've chosen as well as how many groups (*sets*) of those reps. For example, if you have chosen squats as an exercise to do for your legs, I may ask you to do 1 set of 8 to 10 repetitions. After you've chosen your favorite exercises for your legs and other body parts, go to your personal *Exercise Program Chart* (Appendix A) and start filling in your workout program goals. Warming up and stretching out your leg muscles (see Chapter 3 for tips on warming up and stretching) enhances the performance of these muscles and decreases potential strains to your lower back.

Working Your Legs

Fred Flinstone knew something that many of us take for granted: Strong legs can take you many places. Fred and Barney got some serious exercise by powering their cars with their muscular legs. You may not use your legs to power the car you drive, but you still need strong legs to help you jump out of bed in the morning and carry your body weight around each day. Whether you want to ride a bike, jog, run, or just walk to where you're going, having strong legs gets you further — and there faster. Yabba-dabba-doo!

The muscles of your legs are made up of four major muscle groups (shown in Figure 13-1): the quadriceps, hamstrings, gastrocnemius and soleus, and tibialis anterior. The *quadriceps* (also known as the quads) are the largest group of muscles in your body and are made up of four individual muscles that are responsible for extending your lower leg. Think about kicking a ball or climbing stairs. When you kick, your quads provide the power to extend your leg forward. When you climb the stairs and your legs get a little tired and jiggly, you know you are working your quads.

The *hamstring* muscles (hams) oppose the quads, and their most important action is to help you pull your heel up to the back of your thigh. The hamstrings pull you along when you have to run away from the mean neighborhood dog. An easy way to remember these two main leg muscle groups is: Quads push and hamstrings pull. By strengthening these push and pull muscles equally, you help prevent injury to your knee joints and increase your stamina in cardiovascular activities.

The *gastrocnemius* and the *soleus* (calves) are the two major muscles that make up your calf. Combined, these muscles help you tiptoe through the tulips, tiptoe into the house when you come home past your curfew, or simply lift yourself up on your toes so you feel taller. The tibialis anterior (tibia) resides in the front of your lower leg and is referred to as the shin muscle. If you've ever been kicked there, you definitely know where it is. The tibialis works to lift up the ball of your foot and to dig your heel into the ground. When you walk, hike, or run down a hill, you're exercising your tibialis because your heels hit the ground before the ball of your foot. During this downhill movement your tibialis is contracting to help you keep your balance. If you don't perform this sort of exercise regularly, your shins are usually quite sore the next day.

The following exercises allow you to work your legs.

Quadriceps

- Squats
- Double-leg extension

Hamstring

- One-legged lying heel press
- One-legged heel curl

Gastrocnemius and Soleus

- First-position heel raises
- Single-heel raises

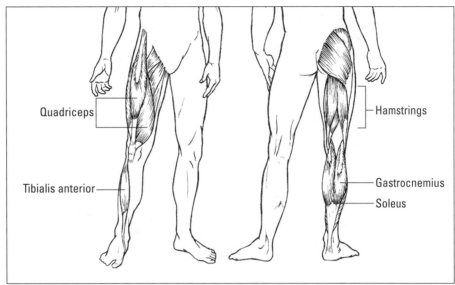

Quadriceps

Tibialis anterior

Hamstrings

Gastrocnemius

Soleus

Figure 13-1:
The many
muscles of
your legs.

Tibialis Anterior

✔ Foot taps side to side

✔ Ankle circles

Simply squats

Women and men in many cultures squat, rather than sit, to work. If you look at Figure 13-2, you notice that in this exercise you don't go all the way down to the floor. In fact, I would like you to check your form in a mirror to make sure your knees don't extend past your toes as you lower yourself down. The incorrect form is also shown in Figure 13-2.

1. **Stand with your feet hip-width apart (perhaps holding on to something for balance and support, like the back of a chair or a broomstick).**

2. **Slowly lower your body downward by pushing your glutes (buns) backward. Think of it as sitting down in a chair.**

3. **Push your weight back up by pressing from your heels, and extend your body up to your starting position.**

Deconditioned Exerciser	Conditioned Exerciser
Sets = 1	Sets = 3
Reps = 8 to 10	Reps = 10 to 12
Weights = 0 to 3 lbs (0 to 1.4 kg)	Weights = 5 to 10 lbs (2.3 to 4.5 kg)
Tips: Place a chair under your buns and lower yourself down as far as you can. If you lose your balance, you have something to sit in. Increase sets and reps after 6 weeks.	*Tips:* Try to hold the squat position for 5 to 10 seconds.

Caution: Be careful that your knees do not bend forward over your toes. Your knees should not extend past a 90-degree angle. Tighten your abdominals to support your torso as you execute the motion. Keep the weight of your body in your heels to work your glutes along with your legs.

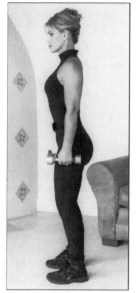
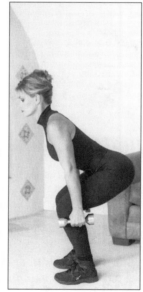
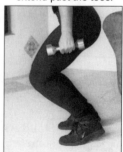

This form is incorrect because the knees extend past the toes.

Figure 13-2: Squats: Not the most flattering position, but great for your legs.

Double-leg extension

Double-leg extensions may not be your idea of a pleasurable experience, but they help you strengthen your legs. Figure 13-3 shows me using a dumbbell to increase the intensity of this exercise. If you're just beginning to work out, feel free to do the exercise without added weight, or if your legs feel strong, you may want to increase the weight.

1. Sit near the edge of a chair or a couch with your hands holding the seat and your feet barely touching the floor.

2. Place a dumbbell between your feet, squeezing your feet together to hold it in place.

3. Slowly extend both knees, taking your feet straight out and up.

4. Squeeze your quads at the top of the motion and then release your legs to their starting position.

Deconditioned Exerciser	*Conditioned Exerciser*
Sets = 1	Sets = 3
Reps = 8 to 10	Reps = 10 to 12
Weights = 0 to 3 lbs (0 to 1.4 kg)	Weights = 5 to 8 lbs (2.3 to 3.6 kg)
Tips: Increase sets and reps after 6 weeks.	*Tips:* Change your count to lift feet up in 3 seconds and resist down in 1 second.

Caution: Work slowly and with control throughout the exercise. Maintain a straight torso with your abs pulled in to support your back. If you have any previous knee injuries and feel pain in your kneecaps when doing this exercise, discontinue it and choose another that is more comfortable for you.

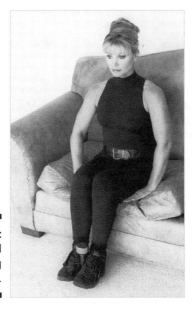 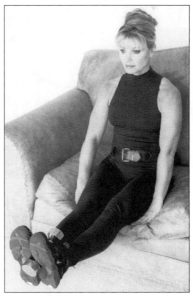

Figure 13-3: Your typical double-leg extension.

One-legged lying heel press

I look pretty comfy in the photo shown in Figure 13-4, don't I? This is an exercise I like to do while watching TV. I can actually make this a "two for one" exercise because, as I press my body weight up from my heel on the floor, I'm exercising my hamstring muscles as well as tightening my buns. If you're not ready for the one-legged version of this exercise, you can try the beginner version (also shown in Figure 13-4). In this case, you leave both of your heels on the floor and press up from both in order to lift yourself off the floor. After you feel comfortable with this position, try the next level, which is described here.

1. **Lie on your back with your knees bent and feet on the floor.**

2. **Cross one ankle over the opposite knee so that the foot on the floor supports the weight of your body.**

3. **Slowly lift your buns off the floor by pushing your hips up from the heel based on the floor.**

4. **Lower yourself back down without resting completely on the floor.**

5. **Repeat and then switch legs.**

Deconditioned Exerciser	Conditioned Exerciser
Sets = 1	Sets = 3
Reps = 8 to 10 each leg	Reps = 10 to 12 each leg
Tips: To decrease difficulty, bring the heel that is on the floor closer to your body. Increase sets and reps after 6 weeks.	*Tips:* Hold your lift for 3 seconds and then release.

Caution: Keep your foot (the one that is based on the floor) flexed. Make sure your hips are aligned with your spine. Tighten your abdominals and keep your back straight. Your hips and lower back should be elevated off the floor at the top of the movement, but your upper back and shoulders remain on the floor at all times.

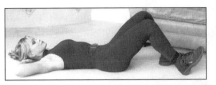
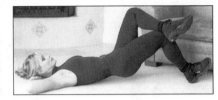
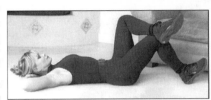

Figure 13-4:
An exercise to do while watching your favorite TV show.

One-legged heel curl

This traditional hamstring exercise (Figure 13-5) helps you develop strong legs, but may make you look like a stork waiting to pick up the next bundle of joy. You can increase the difficulty of this exercise not by holding a baby in your arms, but by adding some resistance (like strapping on an ankle weight or placing an exercise rubber band around both of your ankles and following the steps given here). I show you more about exercising with a rubber band in Chapter 16.

1. **Stand on one leg with the other leg extended behind you.**

2. **Bend your knee so that your foot comes up behind you and slowly lift your heel up to your buns.**

3. **Bring your foot back to the floor slowly and repeat.**

4. **Switch legs and continue the exercise using your other leg.**

Deconditioned Exerciser	*Conditioned Exerciser*
Sets = 1	Sets = 3
Reps = 8 to 10 each leg	Reps = 10 to 12 each leg
Tips: Hold on to a chair for support. Increase sets and reps after 6 weeks.	*Tips:* Add resistance like ankle weights or a rubber band. Change your count to lift up in 3 seconds and resist down in 1 second.

Caution: Be sure to keep the knee of your supporting leg (the one you are balancing yourself on) slightly bent. Don't lock your knee joint. Squeeze your hamstrings and your buns as you contract your leg so that you don't lean forward. Maintain alignment of your head, shoulders, and hips with your supporting leg.

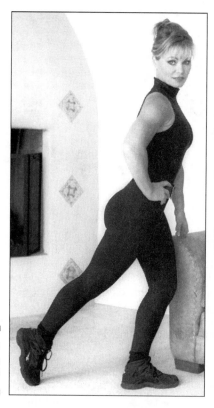
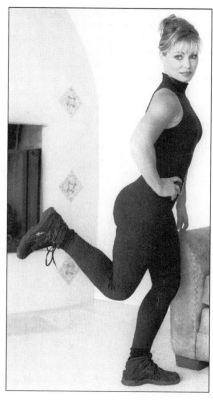

Figure 13-5:
Legs like a
stork, right?

Lifting up to stronger calves

Those of you who have taken ballet classes know this position (first
postion) well. If not, check out Figure 13-6. All you have to do is stand tall
with your feet together and heels touching, and then lift yourself up onto the
balls of your feet.

1. **Stand with your heels touching and toes angled outward at a
   45-degree angle.**

2. **Slowly raise your body weight to the balls of your feet.**

3. **Squeeze your calves at the top of your lift and then release your leg
   to the floor.**

Deconditioned Exerciser	*Conditioned Exerciser*
Sets = 1	Sets = 3
Reps = 10 to 12	Reps = 15 to 20

Deconditioned Exerciser	Conditioned Exerciser
Tips: Do more if you find them easy. Increase sets and reps after 6 weeks.	*Tips:* Hold a dumbbell in your hands to increase resistance.

Caution: Keep your knees straight and work strictly through your ankles and feet. Don't rock back and forth from your heels to your toes. Control your movement.

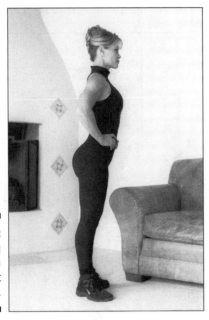 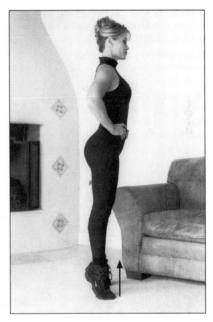

Figure 13-6: Pretending you're a ballet dancer.

Single-heel raises

Next time you are standing in line at the grocery store or maybe the bank, do a few heel raises (shown in Figure 13-7) to exercise your calves. You won't feel like you're wasting time if you have something to do while you're waiting!

1. **Stand on one foot with the other foot resting behind the supporting leg.**

2. **Slowly raise your body weight onto the ball of the supporting foot.**

3. **Squeeze the calf at the top of the lift then release back down to the floor.**

4. **Repeat using your other leg.**

Deconditioned Exerciser	Conditioned Exerciser
Sets = 1	Sets = 3
Reps = 8 to 10 each leg	Reps = 10 to 12 each leg
Tips: Support your balance by holding on to a chair for support. Increase sets and reps after 6 weeks.	*Tips:* Hold a heavy dumbbell in your hands to increase resistance.

Caution: Don't bounce through the motion. Keep your supporting leg straight, but not locked, during the exercise.

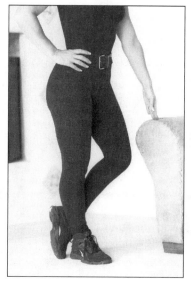 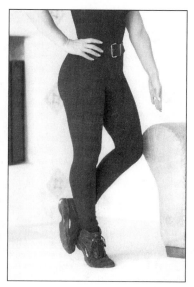

Figure 13-7: An exercise to do while standing in line!

Foot-tapping fun

Strengthen your shins by tapping to your favorite tune, as shown in Figure 13-8.

1. **Sit on a chair with your feet hip width apart and your back straight.**

2. **Lift the balls of both feet up (while keeping your heels on the ground) and move them from one side to the other.**

3. **Concentrate on tightening up your tibialis (shin) muscles by bringing your foot in toward your shin as you lift from one side to the other.**

Deconditioned Exerciser	Conditioned Exerciser
Sets = 1	Sets = 2
Reps = 8 each leg	Reps = 10 each leg
Tips: Increase sets and reps after 6 weeks.	*Tips:* Place something weighted on the top of your feet to increase resistance.

Caution: Make sure you move your feet through the full range of motion. Be sure the movement comes from your ankles and feet — not your knees and hips.

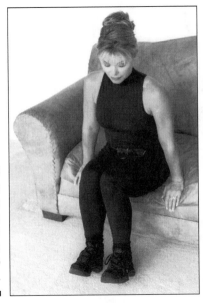 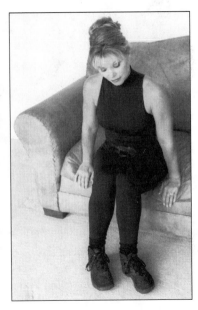

Figure 13-8: You're exercising even when you're tapping to music.

Ankle circles

Here's another exercise you can do while you're waiting or sitting at your desk. You can cross your legs, like the example in Figure 13-9, and start circling your ankle in one direction — then head your toes in the other direction.

1. **Sit in a chair with one leg crossed over the other.**

2. **Slowly rotate your foot in circles (in both directions) by contracting your lower leg muscles.**

Deconditioned Exerciser	Conditioned Exerciser
Sets = 1	Sets = 2
Reps = 10 each leg	Reps = 10 each leg
Tips: Increase sets and reps after 6 weeks.	
Caution: Make big, full circles with your foot.	

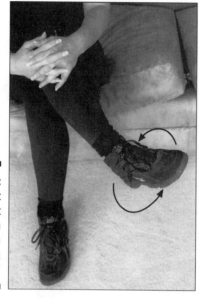

Figure 13-9:
You can get
a workout
even when
you're
sitting
"properly."

Chapter 14

I Love My Thighs: Inner and Outer Thigh Exercises

In This Chapter

▶ Discovering the functions of your thigh muscles

▶ Determining your sets and repetitions

▶ Avoiding mistakes while exercising your thighs

I've decided to dedicate an entire chapter to your thighs. For some women, this may be a blessing. Men aren't necessarily eager to work their thighs for the same reasons as women, but they, too, have a desire to exercise these particular leg muscles. Through the years, I have found the stereotype to be simple: Men want to bulk up their thighs and women want to slim down theirs. Whatever your goal is, you can find exercises in this chapter to get your thighs in shape and discover why these muscles are an important part of your legs' functions. If you are a beginning exerciser, you can follow my recommended numbered of repetitions (reps) of each exercise for the deconditioned person. If you're not sure what your fitness level is, first take a look at Chapter 8 and complete the *Home Fitness Evaluation*. This evaluation helps guide you in creating the best workout for your body. From there, you can choose your favorite exercises from this chapter and highlight them in your personal *Exercise Program Chart* (found in Appendix A). Now all you have to do to get started is to warm up and stretch your muscles (see Chapter 3).

Thinking about Your Thighs

"I hate my thighs." Most women make this statement at one time or another. What these women really hate is the fat that surrounds their thigh muscles. Believe it or not, the jiggle in your thighs doesn't necessarily mean your muscles are weak, but more likely means that you have fat on top of the muscle. Men, on the other hand, usually never experience this "saddlebag syndrome" due to their genetic makeup. It's like a genetic joke on women.

Ha, ha. I know my thighs don't find it funny. Although it may seem that men have it made and don't need to work their thigh muscles to fight the saddlebags, they do need to exercise them to increase the strength of these muscles. Strong inner and outer thigh muscles are critical for changing direction in sports and are frequently injured in various strength and speed sports.

Whether you were born with great thighs or are fighting the saddlebag syndrome, you need to include toning exercises for your thighs in your workout program. The basic exercises in this chapter can help you keep your thighs fit.

Can you get skinny, lean thighs by simply doing 100 leg lifts or "thigh squeezes" every day? Sorry — this is a myth kept alive by false advertising. The bad news is that you *can't* spot reduce body parts, but the good news is that you *can* condition and tone specific parts. For example, if you want to shape up and lose the excess fat in your thighs, you can do toning exercises (like the ones listed in this chapter) that help shape the muscle — but this does not spot reduce or instantly diminish the fat. To really *reduce* the fat in this area, you need to decrease your total daily caloric intake — or to put it simply, eat a low-fat diet. So don't plan on getting rid of fat by exercising your thighs until you can't walk, because you can't eliminate fat surrounding a muscle by overexercising the muscle. On the other hand, if you think you have "thunder thighs" due to excessive muscle bulk, you can reduce the bulk by eating a safe, nutritious diet and increasing your cardiovascular exercise. Toned, lean thighs develop when you combine a nutritious diet with a smart exercise program.

The Ins and Outs of Your Thigh Muscles

Your inner and outer thigh muscles (shown in Figure 14-1) are called *adduc*-tors and *ab*ductors, respectively. The muscles that extend along the inside of your thigh are your adductors, or inner thighs, and help you bring your legs toward the midline of your body. The easiest way to remember what your *add*uctors do is to think about *add*ing your legs together. The muscles along the outside of your hips and thighs are your abductors, or outer thighs, and they do just the opposite of the adductors by pulling your legs away from the center of your body. Both of these muscles help you to keep your balance while riding a bike or horse, or when you ski and skate. Strong thighs also give you greater ability to change directions in sports like tennis and volleyball, and help you to transfer your weight in golf, baseball, and boxing. Have you ever tried to walk on ice? If you're the person who continually falls on your butt or falls down spread eagle, you probably need to work a bit on your adductor and abductor muscles.

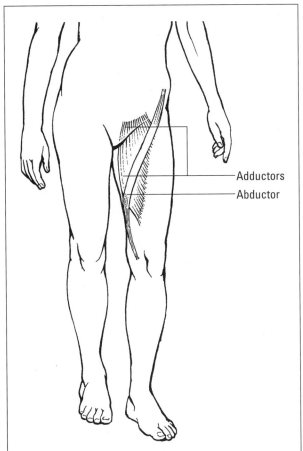

— Adductors
— Abductor

Figure 14-1:
The thigh
muscles.

The following exercises work your thighs:

Adductors

✔ Inner-thigh side lifts

✔ Scissors

✔ Pliés (pronounced plee-a)

Abductors

✔ Lying side leg lifts

✔ Standing side leg lifts

Inner-thigh side lifts (or Adductors Anonymous)

This exercise has been around for a long time and it still works. Figure 14-2 demonstrates a basic inner-thigh leg lift. You'll get a workout by just concentrating on squeezing your adductor muscles as you lift your leg, but if you want to increase the intensity of this exercise, place an ankle weight on the leg you are lifting.

1. **Lie on your side and first place your top leg behind the bottom leg (which is fully extended); keep this knee bent and place your foot on the floor.**

2. **Either prop yourself up on one elbow or extend your arm and rest your head on that arm.**

3. **Lift the foot of your bottom leg (which is straight) and raise it toward the ceiling, then slowly lower it to the floor.**

4. **Repeat using your other leg.**

Deconditioned Exerciser	*Conditioned Exerciser*
Sets = 1	Sets = 3
Reps = 8 to 10 each leg	Reps = 15 to 20 each leg
Tips: Increase sets and reps after 6 weeks.	*Tips:* Add an ankle weight on your lifting leg to increase difficulty.
Caution: Don't swing your leg up and down. Make your movements slow and controlled. Lift your heel up toward the ceiling to focus on adductor muscles. Keep your abdominals tight as you lift your leg.	

Scissors

In the game rock-paper-scissors, the scissors cut up paper, but the scissors exercise (shown in Figure 14-3) can shape up your inner thighs.

1. **Lie on your back, extend your legs to the ceiling, and separate them.**

2. **Place your hands behind your lower back for support.**

3. **Begin with your legs separated as far as you feel comfortable and point your toes up and away from the center of your body.**

4. **Pull both legs in and squeeze them together as they cross the center of your body.**

5. **Release and repeat.**

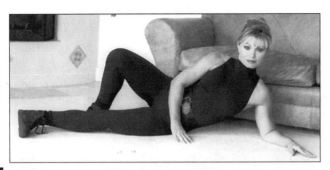

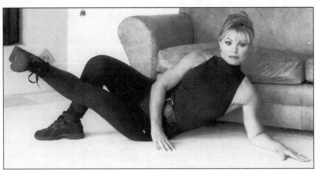

Figure 14-2: Choose a position that is most comfortable for you while you exercise your inner thighs.

Deconditioned Exerciser	Conditioned Exerciser
Sets = 1	Sets = 3
Reps = 10 to 12	Reps = 15 to 20
Tips: Keep your movements slow and controlled. Increase sets and reps after 6 weeks. Place a pillow under your hips for additional support.	*Tips:* Add ankle weights to both legs to increase difficulty.

Caution: Keep your legs flexed at a 90-degree angle to your torso, and don't arch your back. Keep your abdominals tight to support your lower back.

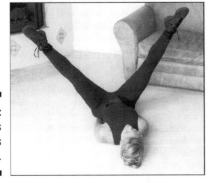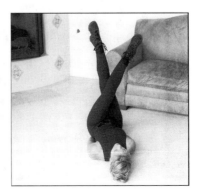

Figure 14-3: A scissors that cuts air.

Pliés

It's not time for ballet class, so don't get yourself stressed about putting on toe shoes to do your pliés. The plié exercise you see in Figure 14-4 is just like the squat exercise in Chapter 13 — except in this one your knees and feet face outward at about a 45-degree angle. This posture changes the focus of the exercise to your inner thighs. After you have the position, all you have to do is squat down and up.

1. **Stand with your feet wide apart and your toes and knees pointed away from the center of your body to help isolate (or focus on) your inner thigh muscles.**

2. **Lower your body until you feel a stretch in your adductor muscles.**

3. **Press up from your heels to raise yourself. Concentrate on squeezing your adductor muscles as you lift yourself.**

Deconditioned Exerciser	*Conditioned Exerciser*
Sets = 1	Sets = 3
Reps = 10 to 15	Reps = 15 to 20
Tips: Use a chair to balance yourself. Increase sets and reps after 6 weeks.	*Tips:* Hold dumbbells for extra weight resistance. Lower yourself down in 1 second and squeeze up in 3 seconds.

Caution: Do not allow your knees to bend past your toes (a 90-degree angle). You should always be able to see your toes as you lower yourself. Keep your chest elevated and abdominals tight. Make sure your feet are wide apart, especially if you are tall.

The everlasting leg lift

Talk about an exercise that never goes out of style! The traditional leg lift (shown in Figure 14-5) has been shaping up our outer thighs for more years than I like to remember. There is no excuse to avoid this one. You can work your thighs while watching TV, reading a book, or talking on the phone.

1. **Lie on your side with your bottom arm extended to support your head, or lean on your elbow to hold your torso up.**

2. **With your hips and legs "stacked" vertically, slowly raise your top leg to contract your abductors and gluteal muscles (your buns).**

3. **Release and repeat repetitions using your other leg.**

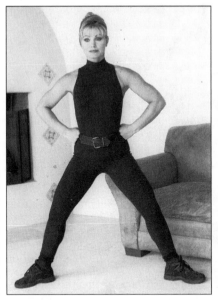 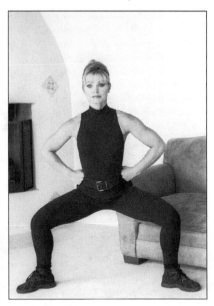

Figure 14-4:
Pliés: an
exercise for
ballet
dancers
and people
like me who
aren't so
graceful.

Deconditioned Exerciser	Conditioned Exerciser
Sets = 1	Sets = 3
Reps = 10 each leg	Reps = 10 to 12 each leg
Tips: You can perform the same exercise standing as an easier option. Increase sets and reps after 6 weeks.	*Tips:* Add ankle weight to your top leg for increased difficulty.

Caution: Keep one leg over the other, don't lean forward or backward, and keep your abdominals tight. Don't use momentum to swing your legs back and forth. Keep your knees and toes pointed forward (foot flexed) throughout the lift so that other muscles aren't recruited to help out.

Standing side leg lifts

Just in case you don't like lying on the floor, I can show you another option to exercise your abductors (see Figure 14-6). If standing is your thing, get your legs moving and give your thighs a workout.

1. **Stand on one leg (base leg) with the other leg just touching the floor with the ball of your foot. The leg barely touching the floor is your working leg.**

2. **Keeping your body straight, slowly raise the working leg outward.**

3. **Release and repeat using your other leg as the working leg.**

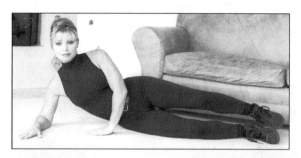

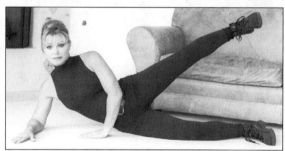

Figure 14-5:
Your
choice:
heads up or
heads down
while doing
your leg lifts.

Deconditioned Exerciser	Conditioned Exerciser
Sets = 1	Sets = 3
Reps = 10 each leg	Reps = 10 to 15 each leg
Tips: Hold onto a chair for balance. Increase sets and reps after 6 weeks	*Tips:* Add an ankle weight to your working leg for increased difficulty.

Caution: Keep the knee of your base leg slightly bent; don't lock up your knee joint. Keep your knees facing forward and your abdominals tight, and lift your legs with slow, controlled movements.

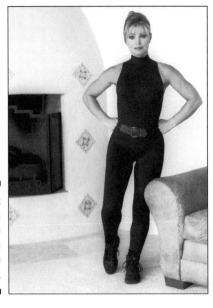 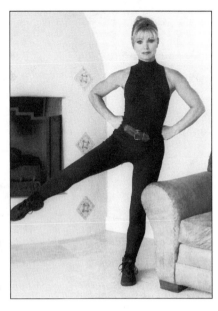

Figure 14-6:
Even when
you're
standing
you can be
exercising.

Chapter 15

Firm Those Buns: Bun Exercises

● ●

In This Chapter

▶ Discovering the functions of your bun muscles

▶ Determining your sets and repetitions

▶ Avoiding mistakes while exercising your buns

● ●

*W*ell, here you are, ready to do my favorite exercises. I try never to teach a fitness class without including a few exercises for the lower half of the body, primarily your buns. My class participants usually approach me a day or two after taking my muscle-conditioning class and have a few words to say to me about the aching in their behinds. Eventually, as they begin to see their bodies firm and shape up, they come back and say thank you to me for being the cause of the pain in their butts.

This chapter shows you what the muscles *behind* you do and gives you some exercises to get them or keep them firm and shapely. If you're not sure whether you should begin following the recommendations for the deconditioned or conditioned exerciser, go to Chapter 8 and fill out the Home Fitness Evaluation. After you determine your current fitness level, you can select the exercises that work best for you. As you can see throughout this chapter, each exercise for your buns has a recommendation for how many repetitions (reps) and groups of repetitions (sets) you should do. You can highlight all of the exercises you choose in your personal *Exercise Program Chart* found in Appendix A. A few key things to remember before you start are to warm up, stretch your muscles, and breathe as you work out (see Chapter 4). If the exercises start to get difficult, holding your breath is not going to make you get in shape faster. In fact, breathing throughout your workout provides your muscles with the oxygen they need to develop. Your buns may be sore the next day or two, but they'll be firm.

TAMILEE SAYS

A bubble butt, my greatest asset!

When I was a little girl, I was teased about my round "bubble butt." Twenty years later, I'm the one who is laughing. I made it a point to keep my bubble butt in shape for the rest of my life (so it didn't turn into a hot air balloon) and now it is one of my greatest assets. It's a bubble butt turned into Buns of Steel!

You're Destined to Have Buns of Steel

I love to work my buns and I've been doing it for a long time. It's probably fate that led me to host the Buns of Steel video series. If you've ever done my buns or leg workouts, you know that you can exercise your buns in a variety of ways — from sitting and squeezing them together to doing hard core lunges and squats. I choose to do them all so that my butt has no chance to get droopy. I want my buns firm and heading north, not sliding down south!

Buns & Associates

LINGO

The largest single muscle in your body is your gluteus maximus (glutes, buns, butt, booty, cheeks, muffins — and the infamous bubble butt), and you're fortunate enough to have one in each cheek (see Figure 15-1). In addition, you also have a gluteus medius and gluteus minimus, as if the maximus muscle weren't enough. The main function of this muscle group is to extend your hip. For example, when you stand up from a seated position, your glutes contract to extend your hip and help you up. Whether you're doing squats, lunges, or climbing stairs, you're gonna be working your buns.

Working your buns requires a lot of knee flexion, so be careful not to overdo it or extend your knees past your toes while doing the exercises. Try to remember not to allow your knees to extend past a 90-degree angle during the exercises.

TIP

The key to maximizing your "maximus" muscles is to keep your weight in your heels during your leg and bun exercises. When you press your weight up from your heels, you can feel your glutes contracting. If you press up from the ball of your foot you can feel the contraction more in your quadriceps (legs).

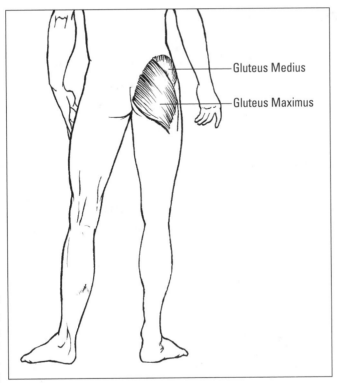

Gluteus Medius

Gluteus Maximus

Figure 15-1:
The gluteus
(bun)
muscles.

Try these exercises to work your buns into shape:

- ✔ Lunges
- ✔ Rear leg lifts
- ✔ Pelvic tilts

TAMILEE SAYS

Hey, I know you.

One day, when Lori (my workout and business partner) and I were traveling, we stopped to check our flight schedule in the airport terminal. I attempted to bend over to search for our tickets, which was difficult due to the mass of people rushing by to make their flights, but I kept getting knocked over. At the height of my frustration, I bent over once more and found our tickets. At that moment I felt a tap on my back and heard a man's voice say, "Hey, aren't you Tamilee Webb, the Buns of Steel girl?" After greeting him I looked over to Lori and asked, "How did that guy recognize me with my head down and my butt in the air?" Being noticed for my butt definitely wasn't one of my childhood dreams.

Bun-burning lunges

Your glutes love when you lunge into this exercise. Looking at Figure 15-2 may give the illusion that this is an easy exercise, but this is one that gets your buns in top form. To avoid any discomfort to your knees and get the most benefit for your buns, pay careful attention to the bend in your knee. The knee of the leg that lunges in front of you should not bend further than a 90-degree angle. The best way to check your form on this is to look down at your foot at the lowest point of your lunge. If you can see your toes, you're okay. If your knee extends past your toes, you need to realign yourself. Try a few and give yourself a break if you get too tired. Just make sure you go back for more.

1. **Stand with your feet together and hands resting on your hips.**

2. **Carefully step forward with one leg and lower your body down toward the floor.**

3. **Keep your front knee aligned over your front ankle and maintain your weight in your front heel.**

4. **Push yourself back to your starting position with your front foot.**

Deconditioned Exerciser	*Conditioned Exerciser*
Sets = 1	Sets = 3
Reps = 8 each leg	Reps = 10 each leg
Tips: Hold on to a chair for balance. Increase sets and reps after 6 weeks.	*Tips:* Hold dumbbells for added intensity.

Caution: Don't allow your front knee to extend past your front toes. Keep a 90-degree angle when your knee is fully flexed. Keep your weight in your front heel to focus on the glutes. Don't bend at your waist; keep your torso straight throughout the movement. Tighten your abdominals to help support your back.

Buff buns

Gear up for some rear leg lifts that lift your buns in more ways than one. You can do this exercise as it is shown in Figure 15-3, or you can make it a bit more difficult by adding an ankle weight to the leg you are lifting. In either case, make sure you don't arch your back as you lift your leg behind you; just concentrate on contracting your glutes.

1. **Stand up straight with your feet placed shoulder-width apart. Place one foot (working leg) behind you. Your other leg remains as your support leg (base leg).**

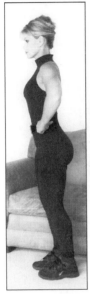 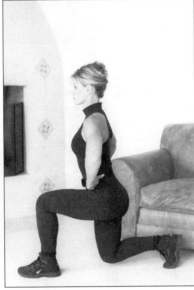 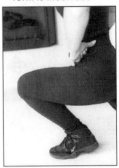

If your knee extends past your toes, your form is incorrect.

Figure 15-2: Love-me-not lunges.

2. **Keeping both of your knees slightly bent, lift your working leg up toward the ceiling without creating a strong arch in your back.**

3. **Squeeze your glutes as you lift and slowly release your leg back to the floor.**

4. **Repeat using your other leg.**

Deconditioned Exerciser	*Conditioned Exerciser*
Sets = 1	Sets = 3
Reps = 8 each leg	Reps = 10 each leg
Tips: Hold on to a chair or couch for balance. Increase sets and reps after 6 weeks.	*Tips:* Add ankle weights for increased difficulty.

Caution: Don't swing your leg. Keep your torso straight and lift your leg as high as you can without arching your back. Squeeze your buns and tighten your abdominals as you lift your leg. Keep your base knee slightly bent; don't lock your knee joint.

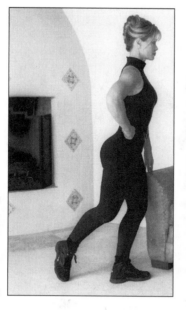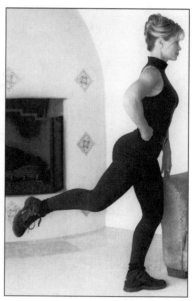

Figure 15-3:
A leg-lifting exercise to elevate your buns.

Couch potato tilts

If you don't have time to work out, but you do have a few moments to watch the news or your favorite sitcom on television, I have good news for you. You can do both. You can easily do the pelvic tilt (in Figure 15-4), a bun-tightening exercise, while you catch up on your TV time.

1. **Lie on your back with your knees bent, your feet flat on the floor, and your hands behind your neck.**

2. **Press your weight up from your heels to elevate your hips off the floor.**

   Concentrate on squeezing your buns together as you move through this motion.

3. **Slowly lower yourself to the floor and repeat.**

Deconditioned Exerciser	Conditioned Exerciser
Sets = 1	Sets = 3
Reps = 10	Reps = 10 to 12
Tips: Increase sets and reps after 6 weeks.	
Caution: Tighten your abdominals as you elevate your hips in order to support your back.	

TAMILEE SAYS

Are you two sisters?

I am very fortunate to be able to travel the world teaching, lecturing, and meeting people from all walks of life. Lori (my workout and business partner) has traveled with me quite extensively and she can attest to some of the crazy questions I get asked. One of my favorites is, "Are you two sisters?" I decided to answer this question on stage when Lori is assisting me with the workout and lectures. I stand next to her (butt to butt) and ask the audience, "Do we look like we're related?" Although you can't visually compare Lori's rear end to mine, if you did, you would know that we didn't come from the same parents. Our body types are very different. I'm a mesomorph (see Chapter 5) with a bubble butt, and she is an ectomorph (see Chapter 6) with no butt. We may have been working and hanging out together long enough to look alike from the neck up, but our bodies always tell our true identities.

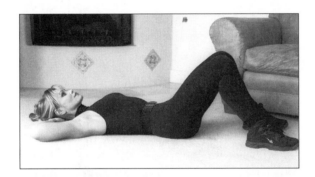

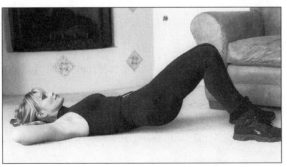

Figure 15-4: An exercise that even couch potatoes can do while watching TV.

Part V
Special Workouts at Home, on the Road, in the Office, or at the Gym

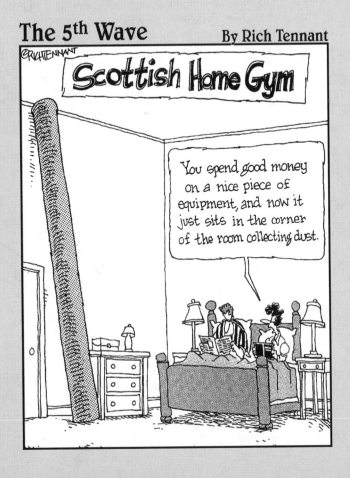

The 5th Wave   By Rich Tennant

In this part . . .

1 have a workout plan that you can do wherever you are. This part shows you workouts and stretches to do while you're in the office or on the road. I also add a special home workout option to do with the exercise band, plus workout programs for older adults and moms to be, and tips for keeping kids active. If you are thinking of checking out a gym, you can find great tips on selecting one that meets your workout needs. I leave you with no excuse to avoid working out after reading these chapters.

Chapter 16

A Home Workout with an Exercise Band

In This Chapter

▶ Working out with rubber bands

▶ Using rubber bands for quick cardio workouts

*T*he rubber band you see in the photos throughout this chapter looks innocent enough, but this little band can give you a tough workout. You can perform all the exercises in this chapter without the band, but working out with a band gives you the benefit of additional resistance. You can mix the exercises in this chapter with your favorites from Chapters 10–15 to add variety to your workout. This little band also makes it easy and convenient to work out while you're away from home. I keep one in my suitcase so I have it whenever I travel.

Before starting a new workout program, I recommend you fill out the Home Fitness Evaluation in Chapter 8, and warm up and stretch out your muscles (see Chapter 4). I list different workouts for either the deconditioned exerciser or the conditioned exerciser to help you gradually achieve your goals.

The Home Rubber Band Workout

"Pumping Rubber," as I like to call it, is one of my favorite workout activities. This product gives me a variety of rubber band exercise equipment to diversify my workouts. I have gotten such great workouts using the bands that I decided to name one of my exercise classes Pumping Rubber and have all my students pump up their muscles with rubber. This chapter focuses on the rubber band itself. If you skip over to Chapter 17, you can find another band workout with the Exercise Bar.

The beginning of bands

I came upon the concept of using a rubber band to get a great workout 14 years ago. I was volunteering in a physical rehabilitation clinic and noticed that the therapists had their patients perform therapeutic exercises with rubber bands. It worked so well, I decided to create my own exercises for healthy individuals. In 1986 I wrote my first book, *The Original Rubberband Workout* (see Chapter 23 for more information). The bands I use for these exercises aren't the typical rubber bands you have stuffed in your kitchen drawer — they're sport bands made from a durable rubber. When I

teach muscle-conditioning classes, I like to mix up my workouts using both dumbbells and bands. The rubber bands provide a *variable resistance.* In other words, the amount of resistance changes throughout the range of motion of your exercise. This differs from a handheld weight like a dumbbell because if a dumbbell says *5 pounds* (about 2.3 kg) on the side, it provides 5 pounds of resistance at every point of the exercise. Try to mix up your workouts. Both dumbbells and bands are great forms of resistance to work your muscles, and the change creates variety in your program.

These workout rubber bands are *almost* indestructible. If you see a tear or a hole in your band, however, don't use it. After it starts to break, you may risk having it slip off or completely split in half.

Leg lifts with a pull

If you looked through Chapter 14, you may have seen an exercise that looks very similar to this one (refer to Figure 14-6 in Chapter 14). The big difference is that I added a rubber band around your ankle to make the exercise a bit more challenging. In order to keep the rubber band from sliding off of the leg you are lifting, you need to flex your foot (pull your toes up toward your shin).

1. **Stand with your feet together and one arm holding a chair for support.**

2. **Keep your knees slightly bent and place the band around your ankles.**

3. **Move your outside leg away from the supporting leg and then back in (keeping your heel angled upward and your foot flexed).**

4. **Repeat on one side and then work your other leg.**

Deconditioned Exerciser	Conditioned Exerciser
Sets = 1	Sets = 3
Reps = 6 to 8 each leg	Reps = 10 to 12 each leg
Tips: Adjust the band to below your knees to make it easier. Increase sets and reps after 6 weeks.	*Tips:* Lift up in 1 second and resist down for 3 seconds.
Caution: Don't allow your hips to rotate throughout the motion. Control the band; don't let it snap your leg back.	

Intensify your inner thighs

This inner-thigh exercise has an added kick. You can't believe the challenge this exercise (shown in Figure 16-1) creates by simply adding a band. You can really pump up the intensity of this one by holding your leg up for a second or two each time you elevate it. After a while, the seconds begin to feel like minutes.

1. **Lie on your side and place your top leg (which should be bent at the knee) behind the bottom leg (which should remain straight on the floor).**

2. **Now place the band around the ankle of your bottom (straight) leg and underneath the foot of your top leg (bent).**

3. **Lift your bottom leg toward the ceiling and lead with your heel, keeping your toes pointed toward your shin.**

4. **Repeat using your other leg.**

Deconditioned Exerciser	Conditioned Exerciser
Sets = 1	Sets = 3
Reps = 6 to 8 each leg	Reps = 10 to 12 each leg
Tips: Try lying on your side, stepping on the band with your top leg, and then lifting with the bottom leg. Increase sets and reps after 6 weeks.	*Tips:* Change the tempo (speed) of the lifts. Increase your reps.
Caution: Keep your foot (which is on the floor) tightly over the band so that it doesn't slip out from under you.	

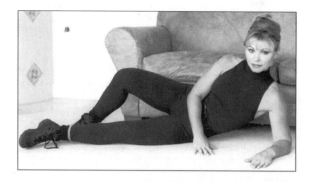

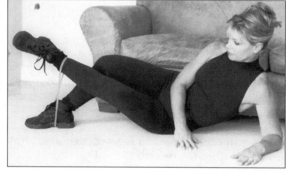

Figure 16-1: An inner-thigh leg lift with a kick.

Seated leg extension

The leg extension is another TV-watching exercise (Figure 16-2), but don't get too relaxed by sitting on the couch. Keep your focus and concentrate on squeezing your quadricep muscles.

1. **Sit on a couch or a chair with the band around the ankle of one foot and under your other foot.**

2. **Keep your foot with the band around it firmly on the floor.**

3. **Extend or lift the other leg forward, straightening your knee.**

4. **As you extend your leg, squeeze the top of your thigh on the same leg.**

5. **Release and repeat, using your other leg.**

Deconditioned Exerciser	*Conditioned Exerciser*
Sets = 1	Sets = 3
Reps = 8 to 10 each leg	Reps = 10 to 12 each leg
Tips: Sit in a chair with back support for greater comfort. Increase sets and reps after 6 weeks.	*Tips:* Lift up in 3 seconds and resist down for 1 second.
Caution: Keep your abs tight on the extension. Don't lock your knees.	

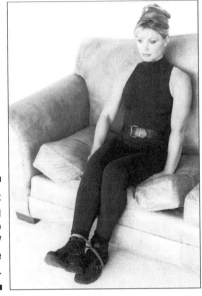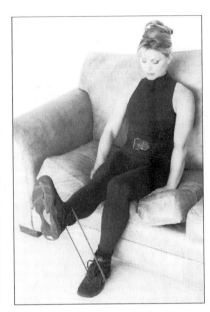

Figure 16-2:
Add this leg extension to your TV exercise routine.

Hamstring curl

This is an exercise (see Figure 16-3) that benefits more than just your hamstrings. If you squeeze your buns, too, you can tone them as well.

1. **Stand beside or behind a chair or couch for support.**

2. **Place one foot behind the other, keep your knees slightly bent, and place the band around your ankles.**

3. **Curl one leg up toward your buns, keeping the foot of the raised leg flexed.**

4. **Squeeze the back of your thigh as you curl.**

5. **Release and repeat; and then work your other leg.**

Deconditioned Exerciser	*Conditioned Exerciser*
Sets = 1	Sets = 3
Reps = 8 to 10 each leg	Reps = 10 to 12 each leg
Tips: Keep your knees together and abs tight. Increase sets and reps after 6 weeks.	*Tips:* Place the band around your foot of the leg that remains on the floor and around the ankle of the leg that you're raising. Lift up for 3 seconds and resist down for 1 second.

Caution: It's best to have socks on or something covering your legs so the rubber doesn't irritate your skin.

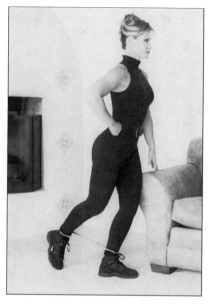 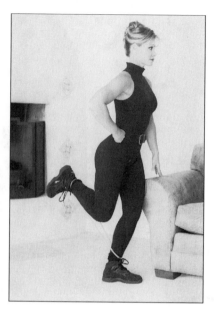

Figure 16-3: This exercise can be beneficial to both your thighs and buns.

Upper-back pullbacks

Figure 16-4 shows an exercise to work the muscles of your upper back. The key word here is *upper*. Keep your arms at shoulder level throughout the movement in order to focus on your upper-back muscles.

1. **Stand with your feet together.**

2. **Hold the band with your palms facing toward your torso, and with both your hands and elbows at shoulder level.**

3. **Keep your elbows at shoulder level as you pull the band, contracting your shoulder blades.**

4. **Release and repeat.**

Deconditioned Exerciser	*Conditioned Exerciser*
Sets = 1	Sets = 3
Reps = 8 to 10	Reps = 10 to 12
Tips: Sit in a chair for support. Tighten your abs. Increase sets and reps after 6 weeks	*Tips:* Increase or decrease the tempo (speed) of your movement. Increase your reps to 16.
Caution: Don't arch your back extensively when you pull the rubber band back.	

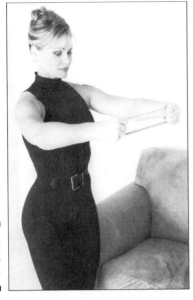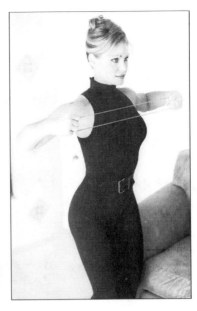

Figure 16-4:
Upper-back
pullbacks.

Overhead pulldowns

The end result of this exercise (shown in Figure 16-5) reminds me of what some guys look like when they are showing off their muscles.

1. **Stand with your feet together.**

2. **Hold the band overhead with your palms facing each other.**

3. **Lower both hands down and out behind your back, pointing your elbows downward.**

4. **Release and repeat.**

Deconditioned Exerciser	*Conditioned Exerciser*
Sets = 1	Sets = 3
Reps = 8 to 10	Reps = 10
Tips: Sit in a chair for support. Keep one arm straight and alternate pulling down each arm. Increase sets and reps after 6 weeks.	*Tips:* Increase your reps.
Caution: Don't bend your wrists; keep them straight.	

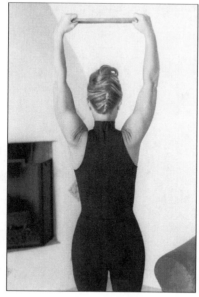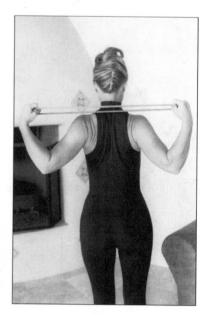

Figure 16-5:
You can show off your great muscles while you do this exercise.

Front-arm curl

How many times a day do you curl your arm toward your face? Add a band, like you see in Figure 16-6, and you can start building your biceps.

1. **Stand with your feet together.**

2. **Hold the band against your right hip with your left hand.**

3. **With your right palm facing up, pull the band up to your right shoulder.**

4. **Squeeze the front of your upper arm as you curl.**

5. **Release and repeat; then do the exercise using your other arm.**

Deconditioned Exerciser	*Conditioned Exerciser*
Sets = 1	Sets = 3
Reps = 8 to 10 each side	Reps = 10 to 12 each side
Tips: Sit in a chair for support. Increase sets and reps after 6 weeks.	*Tips:* Curl your arm up for 3 seconds and resist down for 1 second.
Caution: Keep your wrist straight.	

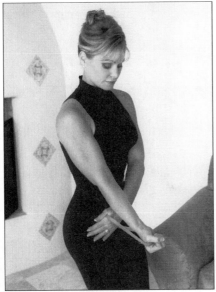 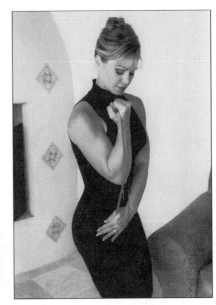

Figure 16-6:
This bicep curl with a band is similar to the exercise you may see people do with weights in the gym.

Working the back of your arm

This exercise (shown in Figure 16-7) focuses on your triceps. Make sure you have a good grip on the band by hooking it around the thumb of the arm resting on your shoulder.

1. **Stand with your feet together.**

2. **Hold the band with your left palm on your right shoulder, hooking it around your thumb.**

3. **With your right palm facing away from your body, press your right hand down to your right thigh.**

4. **Squeeze the back of your upper arm as you press your hand to your thigh.**

5. **Release and repeat the exercise using your other arm.**

Deconditioned Exerciser	*Conditioned Exerciser*
Sets = 1	Sets = 3
Reps = 8 to 10 each side	Reps = 10 to 12 each side
Tips: Sit in a chair for support. Hold your base arm still. Increase sets and reps after 6 weeks.	*Tips:* Press your arm down in 1 second and resist up in 3 seconds.
Caution: Keep your wrist straight.	

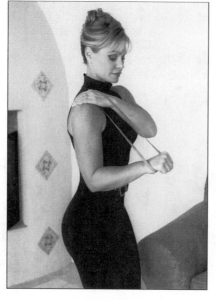 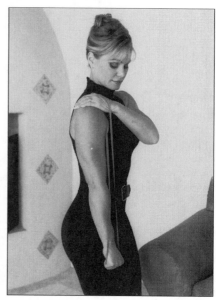

Figure 16-7:
This exercise really puts the focus on the back of your arm.

An intensified abdominal crunch

This is one crunch you'll enjoy. Figure 16-8 shows you how to intensify an ab exercise by adding a band.

1. **Lie on the floor with your knees bent.**
2. **Place the band around both of your legs, between your knees and your ankles.**
3. **With your hands, pull the band from under your legs down to the floor and hold it there.**
4. **Slowly tighten your abs as you lift your chest off the ground and pull your knees toward your chest, keeping the band secure on the floor.**
5. **Release and repeat.**

Deconditioned Exerciser	*Conditioned Exerciser*
Sets = 1	Sets = 3
Reps = 8 to 10	Reps = 15 to 20
Tips: Start with the band around your legs, just above your knees. Increase sets and reps after 6 weeks. Don't lift your chest up; just lift your hips.	*Tips:* Each time you crunch, hold the position for a second or two.
Caution: Make sure you have a good grip on the rubber.	

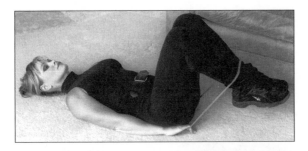

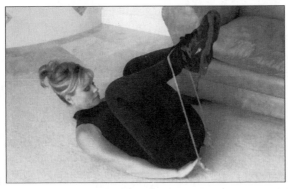

Figure 16-8:
This basic ab exercise is much more challenging when you add the band.

Outer-thigh press out

You may have seen the exercise shown in Figure 16-9 before — and if you've done it, you can probably lift your leg a bit higher. Don't worry about your distance this time. When you add the band, you can feel your muscles working by lifting your leg just a little bit.

1. **Lie on your side on the floor.**

2. **Place the band around your ankles.**

3. **Lift your top leg up toward the ceiling.**

4. **Release and repeat; then complete repetitions on your other side.**

Deconditioned Exerciser	*Conditioned Exerciser*
Sets = 1	Sets = 3
Reps = 8 to 10	Reps = 10 to 12
Tips: Place the band around your thighs for less resistance. Increase sets and reps after 6 weeks.	*Tips:* Lift your leg up in 3 seconds and resist down in 1 second.
Caution: Wear socks or pants that cover your legs so that the rubber doesn't irritate your skin.	

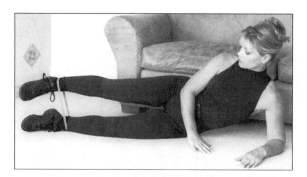

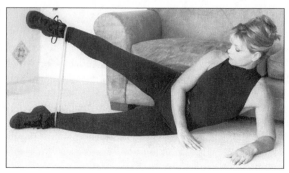

Figure 16-9:
The lift in this exercise is shorter but harder than the traditional leg lift.

Chapter 17
Hotel and Travel Workouts

In This Chapter

▶ Working your muscles with an Exercise Bar
▶ Taking cardiovascular workouts on the road

Most hotels that book business travelers in major cities have some form of exercise room with cardiovascular machines, weight machines, or free weights. You may even find some hotels that provide guests with in-room personal trainers or a selection of workout videos like that excellent series "Buns of Steel with Tamilee Webb." If the hotel you're staying at doesn't provide this type of service, you may want to check with the desk clerk to see if they have an arrangement with local health clubs or a YMCA. Many fitness facilities have exchange agreements with hotels and motels across the country.

If you're lucky to find even an alarm clock as a room perk, or if you prefer to do your own workout while you're traveling, take a copy of the on-the-go workout found later in this chapter.

If you are a beginning exerciser, I suggest you fill out the Home Fitness Evaluation (found in Chapter 8) to determine the best program for you. Chapter 8 suggests programs for both the deconditioned and conditioned exerciser. Before you begin your workout, make sure you warm up and then stretch to prepare your body for the exercises (see Chapter 4).

Don't Tell the Hotel Workout

I'm not secretly trying to put hotel gyms out of business; I simply want to offer you another workout option while you're away from home. I have heard that some people find jumping on the bed a great cardiovascular workout (I won't mention any names). Although I find this to be a fun activity, I know my mother never appreciated it when I was a kid — and I'm sure no hotel manager does, either. You probably want to find a safer and more legal way to get a workout while you're away from home. This chapter provides you with more realistic workout alternatives whether you're staying in a hotel or at a relative's house who does not allow bed jumping.

Another workout option is the Exercise Bar (see Figure 17-1), which is my favorite exercise tool on the road or at home. It's easy to pack and convenient to use just about everywhere. The bar is lightweight and made of wood. You can unlock it and separate the bar into two small pieces for easy packing. All of the exercises in this travel chapter are listed in your Exercise Program Chart (see Appendix A), and most can be done with the bar or with no equipment at all. Bring your chart on the road with you to keep your workouts consistent.

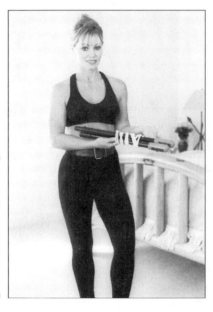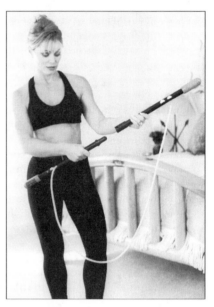

Figure 17-1: No, this is not an infomercial. This is the SPRI Exercise Bar.

Muscle-Conditioning Workout

Many of the exercises listed below incorporate the use of the Exercise Bar, and some can be done just by using your body weight as a form of resistance. If you have a few extras in your hotel room like a chair, a carpet you would consider lying on, and a doorknob, you have what it takes to get a great workout. If you have a chair to work with, try placing the back of it up against a wall or your bed to give it stability. Of course, if you don't have a doorknob, you may want to reconsider where you are staying.

Chair dips

Just imagine that you are about to sit in an imaginary chair placed directly in front of your real chair as you set up for this exercise. You can do chair dips (shown in Figure 17- 2) anywhere you find a sturdy chair.

1. **Stand in front of a chair, facing away from the chair's seat. As you sit down on the edge of the seat, place your hands behind your hips (also on the edge of the seat) and shoulder width apart.**

2. **Lift your buns off of the seat and walk your feet forward so that your knees do not bend past your toes. Slowly lower your body downward, being careful that your elbows don't bend to an angle smaller than 90 degrees.**

3. **Extend your arms, raising your body upward and supporting your weight with your arms.**

   Repeat for the number of sets and reps you have chosen.

Deconditioned Exerciser	*Conditioned Exerciser*
Sets = 1	Sets = 3
Reps = 6 to 8	Reps = 10 to 12
Tips: Bend your knees to a 90-degree angle to begin. Keep your wrists straight. Increase sets and reps after 6 weeks.	*Tips:* When the exercise becomes easy, try using only one arm for these dips. Don't lower yourself so far down that you lose your balance. Straighten your legs out, which is harder than using bent knees.

Caution: Make sure your hands are secure on the chair so that you don't slip off. Keep your chest elevated and head up.

Chair squats

See! There are more ways to use a chair than just to sit in it. You can exercise your legs and buns by squatting in a chair (as shown in Figure 17-3), or try leaning against a wall and imitating the same position of a squat. See how long you can hold an imaginary "sitting in a chair" position while you lean against the wall. It's harder than you may think.

1. **Stand in front of a chair with your feet hip-width apart.**

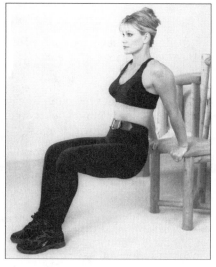 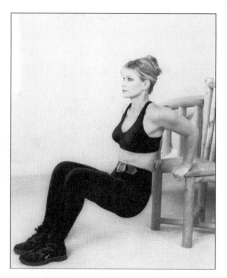

2. **Slowly lower your buns toward the chair without actually sitting down.**

3. **Keep your knees over your ankles and place your weight in your heels throughout the full range of motion. Placing your arms out in front of you may help your balance.**

4. **Straighten your body upright and repeat.**

Deconditioned Exerciser	Conditioned Exerciser
Sets = 1	Sets = 3
Reps = 8 to 10	Reps = 10 to 12
Tips: Keep your knees over your feet. Increase sets and reps after 6 weeks.	*Tips:* Hold on to a light suitcase to increase resistance. Tighten your abdominals. Lower yourself down in 3 seconds and raise yourself up in 1 second. Press your hips forward and squeeze your buns as you stand up.

Caution: Tighten your abdominals to support your back.

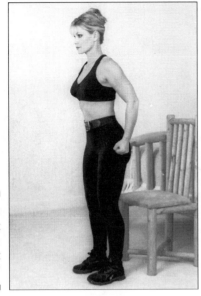 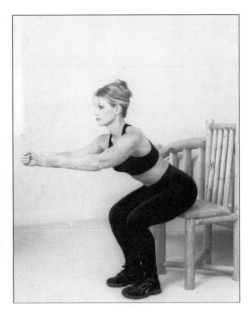

Figure 17-3:
Why sit down when you can just pretend to?

Chair abdominal curls (ab curls)

So maybe the carpet in your room doesn't look like something you want to lie down on. If that is the case, you can still work your abs by sitting in your chair (see Figure 17-4).

1. **Sit in a chair with your hands holding onto the seat and your feet resting on the floor.**

2. **Contract your abdominals by tucking both knees into your chest.**

3. **Lower your legs back to the starting position.**

    Exhale as you contract (tuck) and inhale as you release.

Deconditioned Exerciser	*Conditioned Exerciser*
Sets = 1	Sets = 3
Reps = 8 to 10	Reps = 10 to 12
Tips: Emphasize each abdominal contraction. Just tuck one knee in at a time to make it easier. Increase sets and reps after 6 weeks.	*Tips:* Tuck knees into chest in 1 second and resist back down in 3 seconds.

Caution: Keep your back straight and concentrate on tightening your abdominals as you bring your knees to your chest.

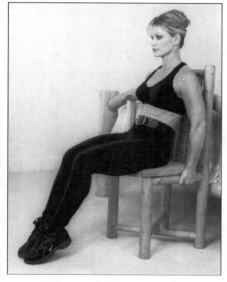 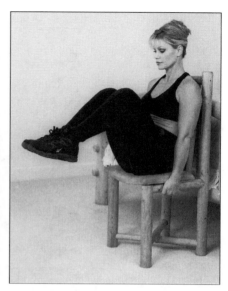

Figure 17-4:
If your carpet has had a few too many guests, try chair abdominal curls.

Iso lunges

This is one of my all time favorite exercises for the legs and buns (see Figure 17-5). You can do it with the Exercise Bar for added intensity or just use your own body weight for a great workout.

1. **Stand with one foot in front of the other. The distance between your feet depends on the length of your legs. Your feet should be wide enough apart so that when you lower yourself your knees don't move past your toes.**

2. **Place your Exercise Bar across your shoulders (behind your neck). The tubing should be under the arch of your front foot.**

3. **Keep the majority of your body weight in the heel of your front foot and the ball of your rear foot.**

4. **Slowly lower your body downward, keeping your front knee aligned above (never extended past) your front ankle.**

5. **Stop the downward movement when your front knee and hip reach a 90-degree angle.**

6. **Return to the starting position and repeat using your other leg.**

Deconditioned Exerciser	*Conditioned Exerciser*
Sets = 1	Sets = 3
Reps = 10 each leg	Reps = 10 each leg
Tips: Hold the bar in front of you at hip level instead. Increase sets and reps after 6 weeks.	*Tips:* Lower yourself down in 1 second and lift yourself back up in 3 seconds.

Caution: Make sure the tube is secure under your foot and that you have a good grip on the bar.

Figure 17-5:
This exercise does wonders for your buns and legs.

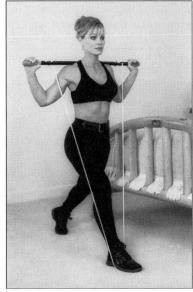 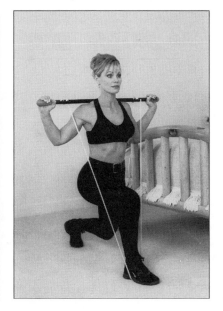

Squats

Intensify your squats by adding the Exercise Bar (see Figure 17-6). If you're really into pushing your limit, you can roll the tube around the bar a couple of times and make this exercise even more difficult.

1. **Stand with your feet shoulder-width apart.**

2. **Place the Exercise Bar across your shoulders (behind your neck) with the tubing underneath the arches of both feet.**

3. **Slowly lower your body downward as if you were going to sit in a chair. Keep your knees aligned above your toes and your shoulders aligned above your knees.**

4. **Stop your movement when your hips and knees reach a 90-degree angle.**

5. **Press through your heels and return to the starting position.**

Deconditioned Exerciser	Conditioned Exerciser
Sets = 1	Sets = 3
Reps = 8 to 10	Reps = 10 to 12
Tips: Separate the bar and hold each handle at shoulder level. Increase sets and reps after 6 weeks.	*Tips:* Lower yourself down in 1 second and lift yourself back up in 3 seconds. Lightly bounce down for 3 seconds and up in 1 second.

Caution: Get a good grip on the bar and make sure it is placed comfortably on your shoulders.

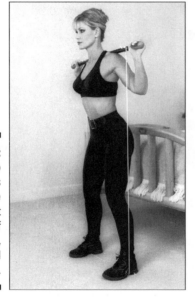 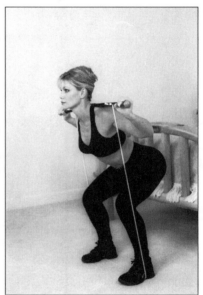

Figure 17-6:
The key to squats is the alignment of shoulders, knees, and toes.

Leg lifts

The exercise in Figure 17-7 gives your outer thighs an exercise they won't forget. Keep your leg straight and add an Exercise Bar to increase the intensity.

1. **Stand with your feet shoulder-width apart.**

2. **Place the tubing under the arches of your feet and hold the bar in front of your legs with your palms facing down.**

   Keep both knees slightly bent.

3. **Lift your leg out to the side, keeping your foot parallel to the floor. Repeat and then alternate, using your other leg.**

Deconditioned Exerciser	*Conditioned Exerciser*
Sets = 1	Sets = 3
Reps = 8 to 10	Reps = 10 to 12
Tips: Separate the bar for less intensity. Increase sets and reps after 6 weeks.	*Tips:* Roll the tube around the bar to shorten the tube and increase the resistance.
Caution: Keep tension on the band with the foot that is being lifted.	

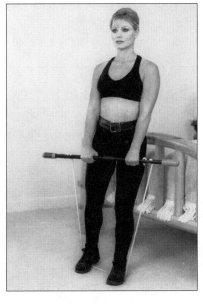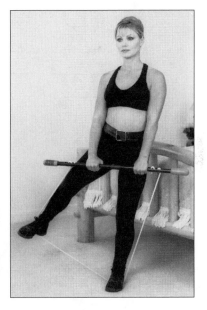

Figure 17-7:
Leg lifts
with a twist.

Back thigh curl

This exercise (shown in Figure 17-8) is just like kicking yourself in the butt — but after you put the tubing around your foot you'll have a harder time actually making contact. Make sure you have the tube placed firmly under the foot you are standing on while you exercise the back of your thighs.

1. **Stand with your feet shoulder-width apart and one foot behind the other.**

2. **Place the tubing under the arches of your feet and hold the bar in front of your body, palms facing up.**

3. **Curl your back leg upward to your buns with your toe pointed to the floor.**

4. **Squeeze the back of your thigh as you curl up.**

   Keep your supporting knee slightly bent.

5. **Repeat and then alternate, using your other leg.**

Deconditioned Exerciser	*Conditioned Exerciser*
Sets = 1	Sets = 3
Reps = 8 to 10 each leg	Reps = 10 to 12 each leg
Tips: Hold the bar lower on your thighs for less intensity. Increase sets and reps after 6 weeks.	*Tips:* Roll the tube around the bar to shorten the tube and increase the resistance.
Caution: Make sure the tube is secure under your foot and is centered under the foot you are lifting.	

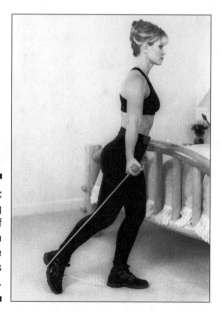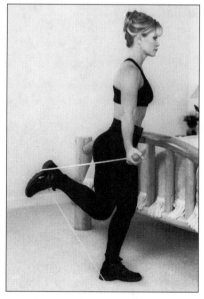

Figure 17-8: Squeezing the back of your thigh during the curl is important.

Shoulder press

Stand tall and impersonate one of the bodybuilders you may have seen on TV. You can do this shoulder exercise (see Figure 17-9) by lifting the Exercise Bar over your head or, if you like, by lifting your suitcase up and over — just make sure you have it closed or you'll end up with a mess.

1. **Stand with your feet shoulder width apart.**

2. **Place the tubing under the arches of your feet and hold the bar in front of your shoulders. Your hands should be shoulder width apart with an overhand grip and your palms facing away from you.**

3. **Press your arms overhead and then return your hands to shoulder level.**

   Keep your back straight and your knees slightly bent. Tighten your abs to support your lower back.

Deconditioned Exerciser	*Conditioned Exerciser*
Sets = 1	Sets = 3
Reps = 8 to 10	Reps = 10 to 12
Tips: Place the tube under one foot instead of both. Increase sets and reps after 6 weeks.	*Tips:* Press the bar up in 1 second and resist down in 3 seconds.
Caution: Keep your knees slightly bent and relax your neck.	

Upright shoulder row

This exercise (see Figure 17-10) makes me think of a butterfly. As you contract your shoulder muscles to lift the bar, your elbows come up next to your ears and create wings.

1. **Stand with your feet shoulder-width apart.**

2. **Place the tubing under the arches of your feet and hold the bar in front of your legs. Your arms should be extended down and your hands placed a few inches apart with an overhand grip.**

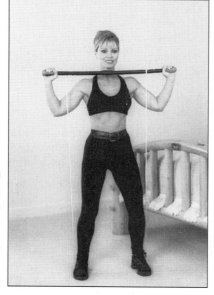 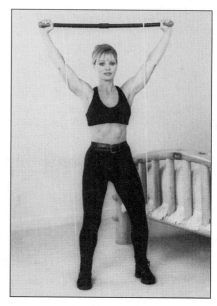

Figure 17-9:
This
exercise
reminds me
of TV
bodybuilders.

3. **Slowly pull the bar up near your chin with your elbows out to the sides. (Hands should reach chin level and elbows should reach eye level.)**

   Keep your shoulders down and relax your neck muscles. Keep your knees bent and abs tight.

Deconditioned Exerciser	*Conditioned Exerciser*
Sets = 1	Sets = 3
Reps = 8 to 10	Reps = 10 to 12
Tips: Place the tube under one foot instead of two to reduce the resistance. Increase sets and reps after 6 weeks.	*Tips:* Roll the tube around the bar to shorten the tube and increase the resistance.
Caution: Make sure the tube is securely placed under your feet before you begin.	

Double upper-arm curl

Have you ever done a chin-up? If you look at the exercise for your biceps in Figure 17-11, you can see that the end point in the exercise looks like you just pulled yourself up over the bar — except your feet aren't dangling in the air.

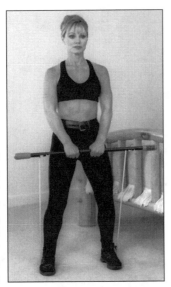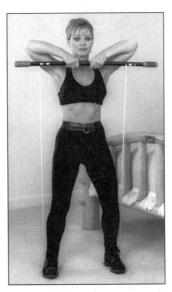

Figure 17-10:
Turn your
arms into
wings as
you build
your
shoulders.

1. **Stand with your feet shoulder-width apart.**

2. **Place the tubing under the arches of your feet and hold the bar in front of your legs with an underhand grip and hands shoulder width apart.**

3. **Slowly curl your hands toward your shoulders and then slowly release them to your starting position.**

   Squeeze the front of your upper arms (biceps) as you curl up. Keep your wrists straight. Keep your knees slightly bent and abs tight.

Deconditioned Exerciser	*Conditioned Exerciser*
Sets = 1	Sets = 1
Reps = 8 to 10	Reps = 10 to 12
Tips: Place the tube under one foot instead of two. Hold your arms closer together. Increase sets and reps after 6 weeks.	*Tips:* Roll the tube around the bar to shorten the tube and increase the resistance. Curl the bar up in 1 second and resist down in 3 seconds.
Caution: Keep the band securely placed under your feet as you curl the bar up.	

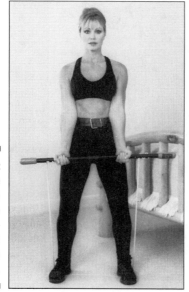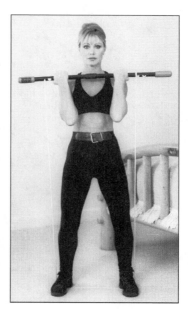

Figure 17-11:
This one looks like you're doing chin-ups instead of bicep curls.

Overhead back-arm extension

This exercise (shown in Figure 17-12) reminds me of the girls in my high school gym class who couldn't throw a basketball correctly (that would be from the chest). Instead they threw it from behind their heads, which is actually working the tricep muscles like this exercise does.

1. **Stand with one foot slightly in front of the other.**

2. **Place the tubing under the foot of your rear leg.**

3. **Hold the bar behind your neck and keep your elbows bent at a 90-degree angle. Use an overhand grip with your palms facing upward, and place your hands shoulder width apart.**

4. **Slowly extend the bar overhead, straightening your elbows, and then release your arms in the starting position.**

   Keep your elbows close to your ears. Tighten your abdominals and keep your back straight.

Deconditioned Exerciser	Conditioned Exerciser
Sets = 1	Sets = 3
Reps = 8 to 10	Reps = 10 to 12
Tips: This may be difficult for beginners, so try a few at a time and increase reps as you feel more comfortable.	*Tips:* Roll the tube around the bar to shorten the tube and increase the resistance. Extend the bar overhead in 1 second and resist down in 3 seconds.
Caution: Make sure the tube is placed firmly under your foot.	

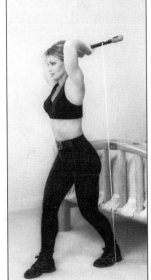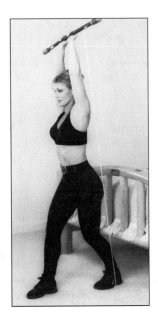

Figure 17-12: This exercise can really make your triceps sore the next day.

Abdominal crunch with the Exercise Bar

This exercise (see Figure 17-13) looks like you're putting yourself into a contraption. It's easier than it looks, and it's really effective in tightening and toning your abdominal muscles.

1. **Lie on the floor with your knees bent and place the tubing under both of your feet.**

2. **Place the bar behind your neck and hold onto it using an overhand grip, with your palms facing your shoulders.**

3. **Curl your head and shoulders upward and your knees into your chest for a full abdominal crunch.**

4. **Release the curl slowly and repeat.**

Deconditioned Exerciser	Conditioned Exerciser
Sets = 1	Sets = 3
Reps = 8 to 10	Reps = 12 to 15
Tips: Eliminate the bar if this exercise becomes too difficult. Place one hand behind your head for support. Increase sets and reps after 6 weeks.	*Tips:* Roll the tube around the bar to shorten the tube and increase the intensity. Crunch up in 1 second and resist out in 3 seconds.

Caution: Wear shoes that make it easy to keep the tube on the bottom of your feet. Bare feet may cause the tube to slide off.

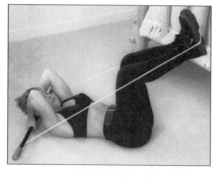 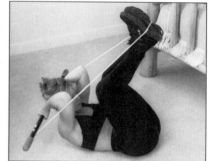

Figure 17-13: Abdominal crunch with the Exercise Bar.

Abdominal side reaches

Imagine that you're stuck between two chairs and you have an itch on your knee. You'll probably bend to the side and scratch it. The exercise shown in Figure 17-14 is just about the same thing, but you are adding a little resistance by placing the tube under your feet and contracting your oblique muscles as you reach from side to side.

1. **Stand with your feet shoulder-width apart.**

2. **Place the tubing under the arches of your feet.**

3. **Separate the bar into two pieces (refer to Figure 17-1). Hold each piece like a dumbbell at either side.**

4. **Slowly reach or slide one arm toward your foot on the same side.**

5. **Keep your knees slightly bent and your torso straight.**

6. **Repeat using your other arm.**

Deconditioned Exerciser	*Conditioned Exerciser*
Sets = 1	Sets = 3
Reps = 10 each side	Reps = 10 each side
Tips: Lower yourself halfway down instead of a full reach to your foot. Increase sets and reps after 6 weeks.	*Tips:* Roll the tube around the bar to shorten the tube and increase the resistance.
Caution: Don't lean forward or twist your torso.	

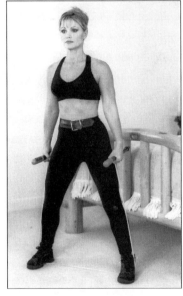 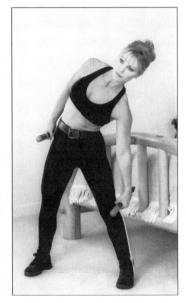

Figure 17-14:
Slide down to scratch your knee or work your obliques.

Lat stretch

Your back muscles get a workout plus a bit of a stretch with this exercise (shown in Figure 17-15). As you lower yourself backward, enjoy the stretch you feel in your upper back and arms. When you pull yourself toward the door, contract your back muscles.

1. Stand facing the edge of the door and place a hand on each knob using an underhand grip. Place your feet shoulder-width apart.

2. Keep your knees soft and drop your hips backward to elongate and stretch your back muscles.

3. Pull yourself back to the starting position and repeat.

Deconditioned Exerciser	Conditioned Exerciser
Sets = 1	Sets = 2
Reps = 8 to 10	Reps = 12 to 15
Tips: Breathe throughout the stretch. Hold for 3 seconds on each set.	*Tips:* Hold for 5 seconds on each set.

Caution: Before you begin, make sure the door is secure and able to support your weight.

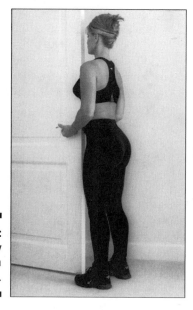 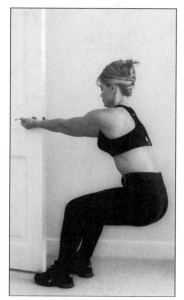

Figure 17-15:
The many uses of a doorknob.

A little extra exercise at the airport

Why are airports laid out like a track and field event? Are the airport people trying to provide us with a means of exercise? Maybe it's just me, but whenever I have to change planes, the gate is always on the other end of the airport. I'm sure some people are entertained by seeing me trip down the halls in my clogs (which, by the way, are not good jogging shoes), rushing to make my flight. As for my luggage, I usually carry it on board with me — which means that as I run from one end of Dallas-Ft. Worth to the other (almost always in my clogs because I still haven't learned my lesson), I get to drag along my rolling luggage and dodge all the poky people as I klipity-clunk by. I admit that once I did catch a ride on one of those annoying beeping shuttles. I wasn't lazy; I was just really late. Actually, I did walk to my connecting flight, which was 30 gates away, and then I realized that they switched the gates (or maybe I read the monitor wrong?), so I had to go backwards 30 gates to where I started. Aren't you tired already? Due to these circumstances, I begged this nice shuttle driver to rush me to the other end. I must admit, it was really fun. So the moral of my mishaps is not that I misread airport monitors but that I can always find a way to get a little exercise in my day, even if I'm wearing clogs!

On the Road Cardio

Your hotel may have an exercise room with cardiovascular machines like treadmills, stationary bikes, and stair steppers, but if not, here are some alternate exercises that can keep your heart strong while you're away from home.

- ✔ Take a brisk walk around the neighborhood or at the local mall. Make sure you take necessary safety precautions before venturing into unfamiliar neighborhoods.

- ✔ Some hotels offer trail maps of their property or the surrounding area. You may want to try a running trail or a hike if weather permits.

- ✔ Check to see if your hotel or local merchant offers outdoor bike rentals and a bike route.

- ✔ Try jogging up and down the stairwell inside the hotel.

- ✔ The hotel may have a pool, or access to a lake or ocean where you can swim.

If none of these appeals to you, stay in your room and do some jumping jacks, or pretend you have a jump rope and get your feet hopping. Whatever you choose, have fun and enjoy your travels.

Chapter 18

Working Out at Work

So you say you don't have time to work out. You're at work eight or more hours a day and exhausted by the time you get home. Your job is stressful and you become even more tense at the thought of having to put another thing, like working out, on your list of things to do. This chapter offers a few solutions for you. Before you say, "No, I don't have any time at work to exercise," give this chapter a chance and try out one of these programs. You can probably complete one of the following office below in 15 minutes or less. Those 15 minutes can help you relieve stress and stay fit and healthy.

I list my suggestions for how many sets and repetitions (number of times you perform the exercise) you should perform if you're a deconditioned or conditioned exerciser. If you find that you can do more repetitions of the "at work" exercises and have the time, take advantage of your opportunity to revive and strengthen your body. Before starting your exercise program, I suggest you do the Home Fitness Evaluation in Chapter 8 and, as always, warm up and stretch first (see Chapter 4 for tips).

Working Out in Cubicle Land

This is the *no time, no equipment workout* you can do while you're at work. All you need is a chair, a desk or table, a nearby wall, and a little privacy if you don't want to show off your newfound "bun squeeze" exercise to your coworkers. You never know — your colleagues may want to join you in the exercise program, and soon your whole office may be doing bun squeezes with you.

TAMILEE SAYS

"Butt Ab US"
(Work your *Butt* and your *Abs* with an *Ultimate Squeeze*)

When people tell me "I have no time to work out," I have to laugh, because you always have time to move your muscles. You may not have scheduled time, so use your down time. If you drive to work, sit at a desk, or lounge on a couch watching television, you have time to do a few Butt Ab US. The time you spend sitting is your down time, and usually averages 20 to 30 continuous minutes, unless you're doing a television marathon. Now, I know you can't throw on cruise control and start lifting weights in your car, but you *can* squeeze your buns while you're driving or sitting in a chair. Turn your radio on, and squeeze to the beat of your favorite music. Squeeze the right and left side of your buns at the same time or add a little variety and squeeze your right cheek, then your left, and then squeeze them both together. At the same time, add an abdominal contraction and continue squeezing your buns and abs for about 20 minutes for a great Butt Ab US workout.

Dipping at your desk

Consider this move just another way to dip into your work. Clear off your desk and take a minute or two to exercise the backs of your arms. Remember to keep your back straight as you lower and raise yourself (see Figure 18-1).

1. **With your hands behind you and shoulder width apart, lean against the edge of a desk.**

2. **Slowly lower your body downward, supporting your body weight with your arms. This exercise looks almost as if you're lowering your body into a chair.**

3. **Be careful not to allow your elbows to pass a 90-degree angle.**

4. **Extend and straighten your arms and then repeat.**

Deconditioned Exerciser	*Conditioned Exerciser*
Sets = 1	Sets = 2
Reps = 8 to 10	Reps = 10 to 12

Caution: Make sure your wrists are comfortably placed on the desk so that they don't slip off easily.

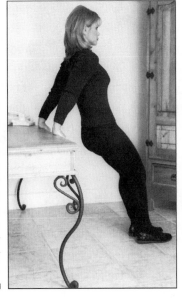 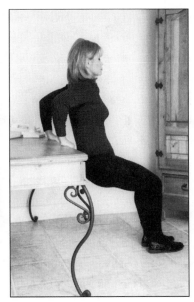

Figure 18-1: The key to this exercise is to concentrate on using your arms to lift your body back up.

Pushing off your desk

You thought boot camp exercises only took place in the military. Think again — Figure 18-2 shows you an option to work your chest, arms, and back by doing desk push-ups.

1. **Stand facing a desk with your feet together.**

   Keep your back straight and your neck aligned with your spine.

2. **Lean forward and place your hands, slightly wider than shoulder width apart, on the desk.**

3. **Slowly lower your body toward the desk and then push away.**

Deconditioned Exerciser	*Conditioned Exerciser*
Sets = 1	Sets = 2
Reps = 8 to 10	Reps = 10 to 12

Caution: Make sure your desk isn't on wheels. Tighten your abdominals to help support your back.

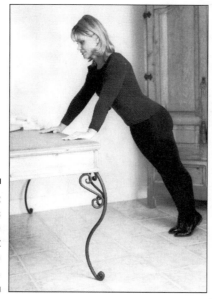 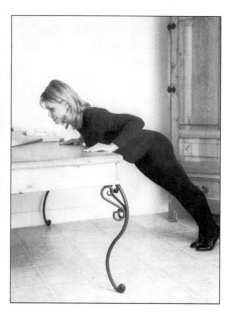

Figure 18-2:
This exercise brings boot camp to your office.

Chair squats

Don't despair; your chair is there if you need it. Figure 18-3 shows you an easy way to work your legs and buns by squatting down in your chair. If you're a beginner, you can more easily keep your balance by placing your hands on the desk and allowing them to slide along the top as you lower yourself. If you get tired, just sit down.

1. **Stand in front of a chair (facing away) with your feet hip width apart.**

2. **Slowly lower your buns toward the chair without sitting down.**

   Keep your knees over your ankles and your weight in your heels throughout the motion.

3. **Straighten and repeat.**

Deconditioned Exerciser	*Conditioned Exerciser*
Sets = 1	Sets = 2
Reps = 8 to 10	Reps = 10 to 12
Caution: Don't allow your knees to extend past your toes.	

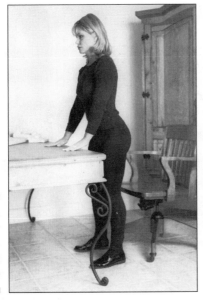 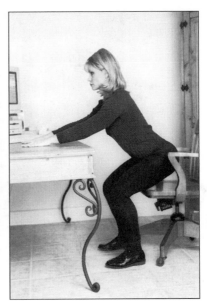

Figure 18-3:
Chair
squats
really work
your thighs.

Leg lifting at lunch

Here is an exercise for your legs that you can do while you're having lunch. Figure 18-4 demonstrates how to work the front of your thigh (your quadricep) by straightening your knee and lifting your foot off the ground. Sit on the edge of your chair with your hand holding onto the edge for support.

1. **Sit on a chair with your feet on the floor.**

2. **Lift one foot forward, extending your knee.**

3. **Squeeze the front of the upper thigh as you lift your leg and hold at the top for a moment.**

4. **Repeat and then complete repetitions using your other leg.**

Deconditioned Exerciser	*Conditioned Exerciser*
Sets = 1	Sets = 2
Reps = 8 each leg	Reps = 15 each leg
Caution: Keep your back straight and don't round your shoulders forward.	

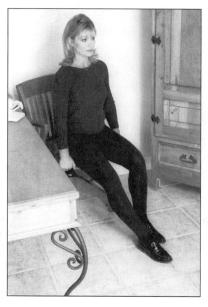 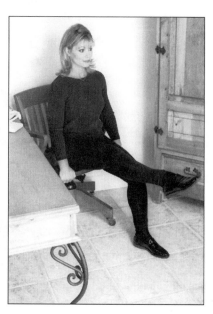

Figure 18-4:
Have a lite bite for lunch and exercise your thighs.

Bun squeezes

You can do this exercise any time you sit at your desk by just squeezing and smiling.

1. **Sit in a chair and squeeze your buns together tightly.**

2. **Hold for two seconds, then release. Increase the speed of your squeezes if you want to increase the intensity.**

3. **Repeat, or alternate squeezing from one side to the other.**

Deconditioned Exerciser	*Conditioned Exerciser*
Sets = 1	Sets = 2
Reps = 10	Reps = 20

Caution: I recommend that you don't do this at important meetings in the conference room.

Up and down, up and down

How much simpler can it be? Just lift your body up and out of your chair several times (like in Figure 18-5) to get your blood circulating and work the muscles of your legs and buns.

1. **Sit on the edge of a chair.**

2. **Stand up, squeezing your buns together tightly and then releasing them.**

3. **Lower yourself back to your chair and repeat.**

Deconditioned Exerciser	*Conditioned Exerciser*
Sets = 1	Sets = 2
Reps = 8 to 10	Reps = 10 to 12
Caution: Watch out for rolling chairs.	

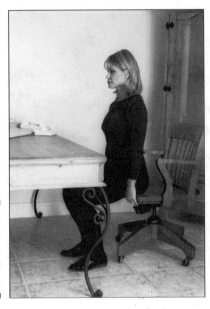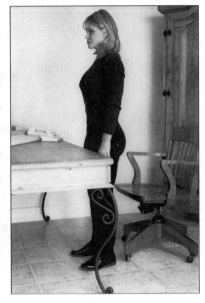

Figure 18-5:
This simple exercise really works your buns.

Toe-ups

Work your calves with the exercise shown in Figure 18-6. It may not look like much, but you can tighten and tone with a few easy lifts.

1. **Stand facing a desk or table, touching the top for balance.**

2. **Place one foot (with your toes pointed on the ground) behind your other heel.**

3. **Raise the heel of your planted foot off the floor as high as possible, pressing through the ball of your foot.**

4. **Squeeze your calf at the top of the motion.**

5. **Repeat, reversing the position of your legs.**

Deconditioned Exerciser	Conditioned Exerciser
Sets = 1	Sets = 2
Reps = 8 to 10	Reps = 10 to 12

Caution: It's best to do this with no shoes or low-heeled shoes for greater comfort.

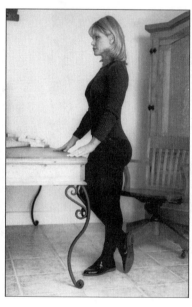 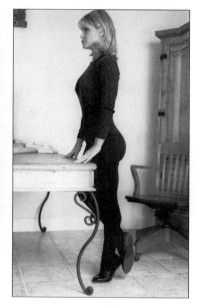

Figure 18-6:
Take a break a few times a day to lift yourself up on your toes.

Tucking it in for tighter abs

Just in case you thought you could abandon your abdominal exercises when you're at work, I'm giving you an exercise you can do at your desk (shown in Figure 18-7).

1. **Sit in a chair with your hands on your shoulders. Your elbows should be at nearly shoulder level on either side.**

2. **Contract your abdominals as you raise one knee in toward your chest.**

3. **Diagonally turn the shoulder that is opposite of the knee you are raising, and connect your elbow with your knee.**

4. **Alternate your legs and exhale as you tighten your abdominal muscles.**

Deconditioned Exerciser	Conditioned Exerciser
Sets = 1	Sets = 2
Reps = 8 to 10	Reps = 10 to 12

Caution: Don't bend your whole torso forward; just turn your elbow toward your knee.

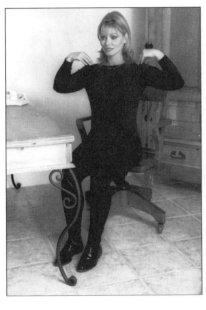 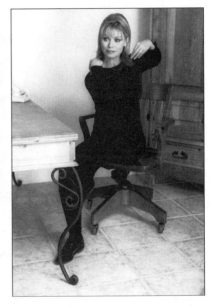

Figure 18-7: Your leg and shoulder make most of the movements here, but your abs are at work.

Picking up your pens

Drop your pen now and then to reach down and tighten the sides of your abdominal muscles (obliques). Just sit in your chair and reach down to touch your ankle (as shown in Figure 18-8).

1. **Sit on the edge of a chair with your feet on the floor.**

2. **Use one arm to reach toward your ankle on the same side, bending sideways.**

Keep your abs in and torso in an upright position.

3. Repeat, using your other arm.

Deconditioned Exerciser	Conditioned Exerciser
Sets = 1	Sets = 2
Reps = 8 to 10 each side	Reps = 10 to 12 each side
Caution: Make sure you're comfortable in the chair and that you don't fall off.	

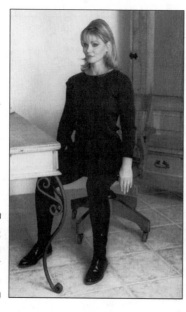 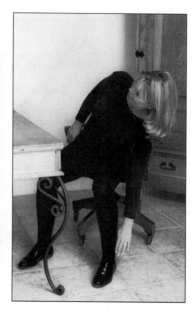

Figure 18-8:
Reaching
for better
ab muscles.

Using Rubber Bands for a Workout, Not Work

The band in these figures may seem like a silly little rubber band, but looks can be deceiving. The band can be stored in your desk, your purse, or your briefcase. Pull it out for a quick workout, or use it as a slingshot if you're bored. If you're interested in purchasing a rubber band or two, check out the coupon included in the back of this book. Have fun, but don't poke anyone's eye out. A helpful hint for women: Don't wear nylons while doing these exercises. Chances are you'll get a run in them after the first few leg exercises.

An under-your-desk thigh workout

Chances are you'll prefer to do this exercise with pants on. Rubber isn't very comfortable on bare skin. Figure 18-9 shows an exercise to help get your outer thighs in shape by simply pressing your legs out. You can lift up your heels and just keep the balls of your feet on the ground if you find it gives you greater comfort.

1. **Sit on the edge of your chair with the band around your thighs (just above your knees). Keep your back straight.**

2. **Press your knees outward, hold for 2 seconds, and slowly release them.**

Deconditioned Exerciser	*Conditioned Exerciser*
Sets = 1	Sets = 2
Reps = 8	Reps = 10
Caution: Control the rubber band; don't allow it to snap your legs back together.	

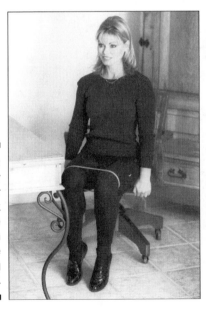 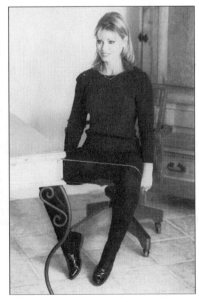

Figure 18-9: Slide your legs under the desk and no one will even know you're working out.

Kick up your heels

This exercise (shown in Figure 18-10) is just like the reflex action you see when the doctor taps your knee and your foot jerks out in front of you. Just make sure you don't kick anyone walking by as you exercise your legs.

1. **Sit on a chair with your feet on the floor.**

2. **Place the band around your ankles.**

3. **Slowly lift one leg upward, extending your knee.**

4. **Release and repeat; then complete repetitions using your other leg.**

Deconditioned Exerciser	Conditioned Exerciser
Sets = 1	Sets = 2
Reps = 8 to 10 each leg	Reps = 10 to 12 each leg

Caution: Make sure you have enough room to bring your foot up as high as you can.

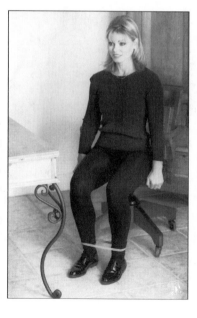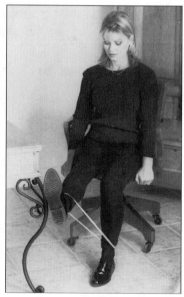

Figure 18-10: You can kick your trash can, but don't kick your boss as he or she walks by.

Standing around brainstorming

You don't have to stop working to exercise your inner thighs. Just brace yourself on your desk and think up brilliant ideas as you kick your heels up (see Figure 18-11).

1. **Stand next to a desk or table for balance.**

2. **Place the band around both of your ankles.**

3. **Lift your leg that is closest to the desk up and across your body. Try to point your heel toward the ceiling, turn your toe outward, and keep your knee bent as you lift your leg.**

4. **Release and repeat; then complete repetitions reversing the roles of your legs.**

Deconditioned Exerciser	*Conditioned Exerciser*
Sets =1	Sets = 2
Reps = 8 to 10 each leg	Reps = 10 to 12 each leg

Caution: Don't get too confused by Step 3. As long as you are lifting your leg and feeling tension in your inner thigh, you're doing fine.

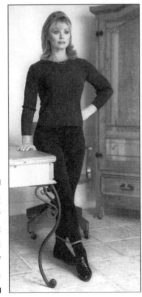
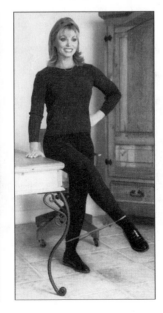

Figure 18-11: Work your inner thighs as you plan for your day ahead.

A break-time back-thigh curl

You may have seen this exercise (see Figure 18-12) before. When you're just standing around, throw your rubber band on and exercise your hamstring muscles.

1. **Stand with one foot behind the other, knees slightly bent, and place the band around your ankles. Use a desk for balance and support.**

2. **With a flexed foot, curl one leg up to your buns.**

3. **Squeeze the back of your thigh as you curl.**

4. **Release and repeat; then complete repetitions using your other leg.**

Deconditioned Exerciser	*Conditioned Exerciser*
Sets = 1	Sets = 2
Reps = 8 to 10 each leg	Reps = 10 to 12 each leg
Caution: Keep the knee of your standing leg slightly bent.	

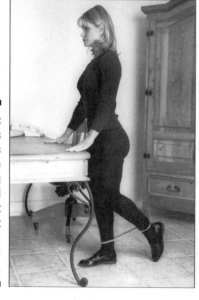 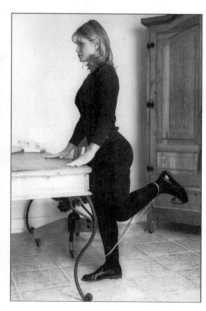

Figure 18-12: This exercise is just like the hamstring curl machine at the gym, but with a rubber band instead.

Re-energize your upper body

You can wake up the muscles of your upper back with the exercise shown in Figure 18-13. Just pull your shoulder blades together as you squeeze your back muscles and stretch the band across your chest.

1. **Sit in a chair with your feet on the floor.**

2. **Hold the band at shoulder level with your palms facing in and elbows up.**

3. **Keep your elbows shoulder level as you stretch the band across your chest and contract your shoulder blades.**

4. **Release and repeat.**

Deconditioned Exerciser	Conditioned Exerciser
Sets = 1	Sets = 2
Reps = 10	Reps = 12

Caution: Keep the band at the same distance from your body throughout the exercise so it doesn't grab onto your clothing.

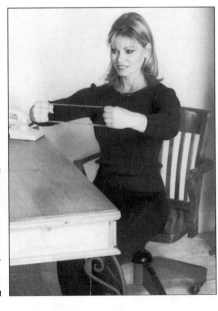 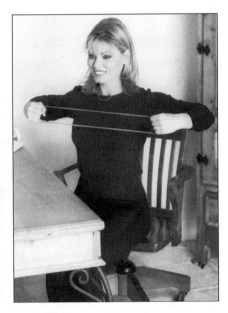

Figure 18-13: This exercise looks like you're taking your coat off.

A pectoral pick-up

Strengthen your chest (pectoral) muscles with the exercise shown in Figure 18-14. Keep your hands directly in front of you and push your palms out as far as you can. Let the rubber band retract slowly so that it doesn't snap off your hands and hit your coworker in the head.

1. **Sit in a chair with your feet on the floor.**

2. **With your palms facing out, cross your arms like an "X" in front of you. When you place the band around your hands, each palm touches the band.**

3. **Press each palm outward with your arms in the crossed position.**

4. **Squeeze your chest muscles as you push out and then slowly release as you allow the band to retract.**

5. **Place the opposite arm on top and repeat.**

Deconditioned Exerciser	*Conditioned Exerciser*
Sets = 1	Sets = 2
Reps = 10 with each arm as the top arm	Reps = 12 with each arm as the top arm

Caution: Don't slouch forward as you do this exercise. Sit up straight and tighten your abs.

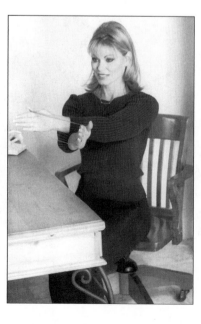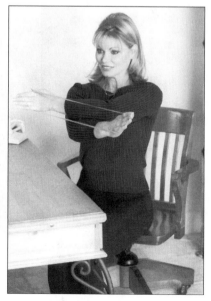

Figure 18-14: You don't have to be double-jointed to do this chest crossover.

Bionic biceps

You need to find a few minutes when you aren't writing or typing at work to do the bicep curl exercise in Figure 18-15.

1. **Sit on a chair with your feet on the floor.**

2. **Use your right hand (with the band looped under your palm) to hold the band to your left thigh. With the other end of the band in your left fist, curl the band to your left shoulder.**

3. **Squeeze the front of your upper arm (bicep) on the curl.**

4. **Release and complete repetitions; then repeat using your other arm.**

Deconditioned Exerciser	Conditioned Exerciser
Sets = 1	Sets = 2
Reps = 8 to 10 each side	Reps = 10 to 12 each side

Caution: Make sure you have a good grip on the band; keep it secure on your thigh so that it doesn't snap up.

Figure 18-15: This exercise gives the tricep muscle on your opposite arm a workout while you concentrate on curling your biceps.

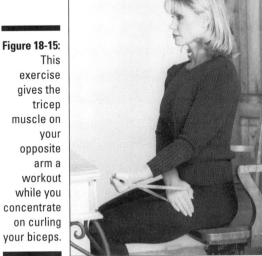
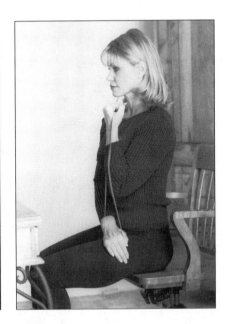

Tightening up your triceps

If you're worried about your arms jiggling as you wave good-bye or write on the chalkboard, you need the exercise in Figure 18-16.

1. **Sit in a chair with your feet on the floor.**

2. **With the band looped around your right palm, hold the band against your left shoulder.**

3. **With your left palm facing away from your body, loop your left hand in the other end of the band and press your left hand to your left thigh.**

4. **Squeeze the back of your upper arm; then release and repeat.**

Deconditioned Exerciser	*Conditioned Exerciser*
Sets = 1	Sets = 2
Reps = 8 to 10 each side	Reps = 10 to 12 each side

Caution: Make sure you have a good grip on the band so that it doesn't snap back at you.

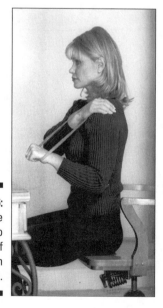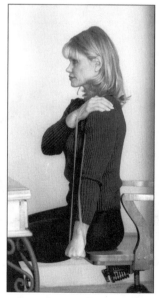

Figure 18-16: This is the exercise to rid yourself of back-arm jiggles.

Overhead pulldowns

This exercise (see Figure 18-17) is like shooting a bow and arrow up over your head. It's a great way to work back muscles and de-stress yourself a bit.

1. **Sit in a chair with your feet on the floor.**

2. **Hold the band overhead with your palms facing in.**

3. **Pull one hand down to your shoulder on the same side. Your other arm should remain overhead.**

4. **Release, repeat, and alternate arms.**

Deconditioned Exerciser	*Conditioned Exerciser*
Sets = 1	Sets = 2
Reps = 8 to 10 each side	Reps = 10 to 12 each side
Caution: Sit up straight and tuck your abdominals in.	

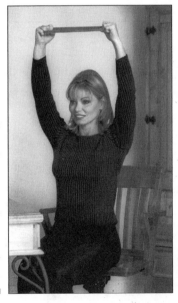 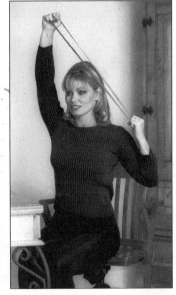

Figure 18-17: This may sound like a good idea, but please don't play Robin Hood by shooting your rubber band.

Tuck in for tighter abs

Give this abdominal exercise a try when you need a break or are bored at the next company meeting (see Figure 18-18). To make this exercise more difficult or more noticeable at your meetings, try a double-knee tuck.

1. **Sit in a chair with your hands holding the seat or arm rests.**

2. **Pull your chest in slightly toward your knees and contract your abdominals as you pull each knee in toward your chest. Alternate pulling each knee into your chest.**

3. **Exhale as you bring your knees toward your chest and slowly relax your abdominal muscles as you drop your knees away from your chest.**

Deconditioned Exerciser	*Conditioned Exerciser*
Sets = 1	Sets = 2
Reps = 8 to 10 each leg	Reps = 10 to 12 each leg

Caution: Start with one leg at a time unless you feel strong enough to pull in both knees at once.

Figure 18-18: A seated abdominal crunch can help you through a tough meeting.

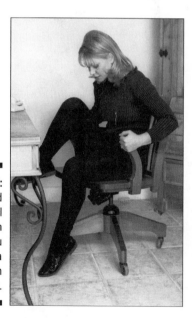
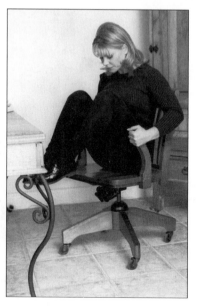

Stretching to Beat Stress

Sometimes all you need is a little rest and relaxation to make it through the day. Incorporate stretches into your workday to keep yourself relaxed and limber. You can repeat these stretches as often as you like. Keep a copy of this stretch program at your desk as a reminder to relax throughout your day.

Neck stretch

This is one you won't mind putting your neck out for. Relax the muscles of your neck by following the stretch in Figure 18-19.

1. **Sit in a chair with your shoulders relaxed, and drop your head to your right shoulder. Hold for 15 seconds.**

2. **Repeat on the left side.**

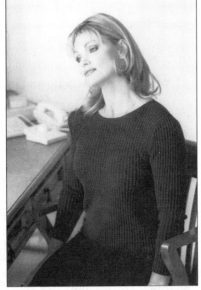

Figure 18-19:
Take a few deep breaths as you loosen the muscles of your neck.

You deserve stress relief

My first job in the fitness industry was at the famous Golden Door Health and Fitness Spa in California. I met people from around the world who came to visit the spa for a little rest and relaxation, and they all came in with a distinctive look about them. Their shoulders were tightened up to their ears, their necks were pulled in like turtles' necks, and they had stress and tension written all over their faces. Most of the guests were only at the spa for 6 days, but each of those days was filled with exercise, nutritious food, relaxing stretches, and lots of laughter. The guests left the spa with a golden glow surrounding their bodies and big smiles on their faces. A spa may not be your thing, but a little R & R is good for everyone. Even if you only take a few moments out of your day, give your body a stretch and take some time to relax and rejuvenate. You DESERVE IT!

Shoulder rolls

This stretch (shown in Figure 18-20) is similar to what your mom may have told you to do when she wanted you to sit up with good posture. You can relax the muscles of your upper back if you emphasize lifting and dropping your shoulder blades as well as your shoulders.

1. **Relax your neck and roll both of your shoulders up and in a *backward* motion 8 times.**

2. **Next, roll them both up and in a *forward* motion 8 times.**

Deltoid stretch

If you happen to be lifting a lot of things or you play sports that require you to swing your arms (like golf and tennis), you'll really enjoy the stretch shown in Figure 18-21.

1. **Cross your right arm across your chest by using your left hand to hold on to the upper portion of your right arm (do not press directly on your elbow). Keep your shoulders down and neck relaxed.**

2. **Hold the stretch for 15 seconds.**

3. **Repeat, reaching with your left arm.**

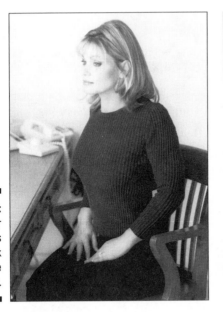
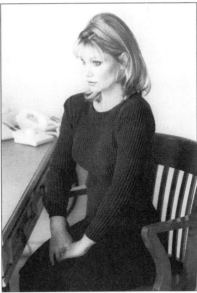

Figure 18-20:
Relax your
shoulders
and back
with these
rolls.

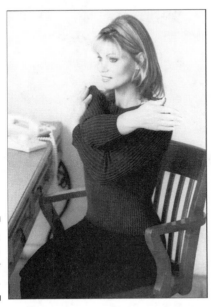
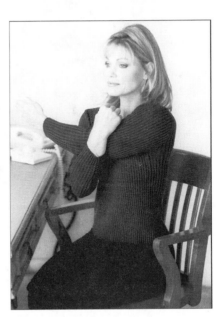

Figure 18-21:
A stretch
for your
shoulders.

Chest stretch

I think we've all done this stretch (see Figure 18-22) at one time or another. If you find yourself slumping at your desk, give yourself a pick-me-up with this chest stretch.

1. **Clasp both hands behind your back at your waistline.**

2. **Keep your head up and lift your arms upward until you feel the stretch through your chest.**

3. **Hold the stretch for 15 seconds and then release.**

Figure 18-22: Put an end to your slumping with this stretch.

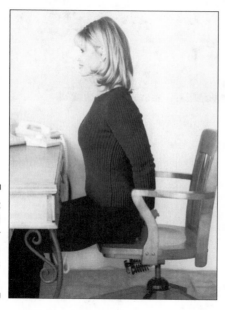 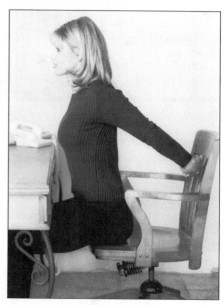

The pretzel

This is not a snack break; it's a break to stretch your back and hips. The stretch shown in Figure 18-23 demonstrates this pretzel twisting stretch, but remember not to turn your body past your comfort level.

1. **Sitting in a chair, cross your right leg over your left.**

2. **Hold onto your knee with your left hand as you slowly rotate your torso to your right side. Hold this position for 15 seconds.**

3. **Cross your left leg over your right and repeat, rotating your torso to the left.**

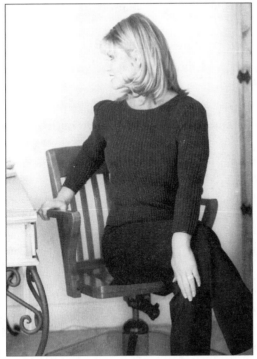

Lower-back knee tuck

Tucking your knees to your chest really stretches out your lower back.
Figure 18-24 shows you how to easily pull your knee up and press out your
spine to stretch your back.

1. **Sitting in a chair with your feet on the floor, lift one knee up to your**
   chest, looping your arms underneath your knee.

2. **As you raise your knee to your torso, pull your abs in and press your**
   back outward.

3. **Hold for 15 seconds and then repeat using your other leg.**

Hamstring stretch

If you can't get your leg completely straight like the stretch shown in
Figure 18-25, start with a bent knee and work towards increasing your
flexibility in the back of your thighs.

1. Sitting in a chair, place one leg on your desk and straighten it out if you can.

2. Lower your torso down to the straight leg.

3. Hold for 15 seconds, and then repeat using your other leg.

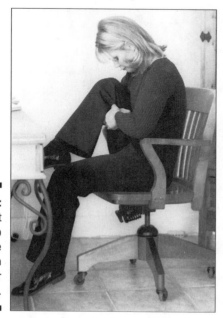

Figure 18-24: A great stretch to release the tension in your lower back.

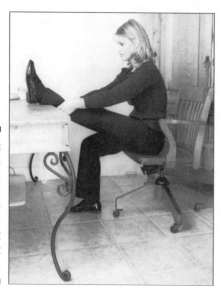 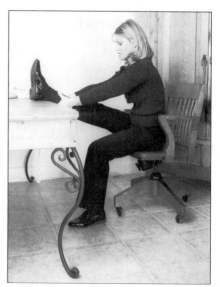

Figure 18-25: This straight leg hamstring stretch is more difficult than it looks.

Side bends

Stretch out your whole upper body with a few side bends (shown in Figure 18-26). Just don't fall off your chair in the process.

1. **Sitting in a chair, place your right hand above your head and reach to your left side.**

2. **Keep your torso straight (no forward flexion) and hold the position for 15 seconds.**

3. **Release and repeat, using your left arm.**

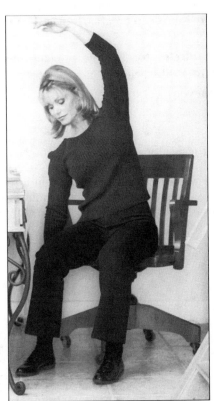

Figure 18-26:
Side bends.

Pumping Up Your Heart at Work

You can find many ways to get your heart racing at work. (Besides, of course, just trying to meet deadlines.) If your office doesn't offer an employee fitness room, check out these options to get a quick workout during your working day.

- ✔ Whenever possible, *don't sit!* If your job requires that you be at a desk most of the day, take a few moments every hour to get up and move around. When you get your circulation going and your blood flowing, you feel more alert and are probably more effective at your tasks.

- ✔ If you have a cordless phone, get up and walk around the room as you talk. If you're stuck with a two-foot range on your telephone cord, do some chair squats while you negotiate your next deal.

- ✔ Try standing at your desk and march or jog in place. (I recommend avoiding this one if you happen to have dress shoes on.)

- ✔ Make it a point to get away from your desk every half hour or hour to visit the restroom, get a glass of water, and do a posture check. When you are seated, sit up straight, keep your shoulders back (not rounded forward), and remember to take deep breaths, letting the tension out as you exhale.

- ✔ Take the stairs instead of the elevator. Try this for eight weeks straight and see how much stronger your legs become!

- ✔ Park your car further from your workplace than you usually do and walk the extra distance.

- ✔ Ride your bike to work.

- ✔ Take a brisk walk outside or in a local mall at lunch.

Any activity is great as long as you are up and moving around. Your goal should be to move your body as much as possible throughout the day. Be creative and design your own workout with the options and equipment that you have.

Chapter 19

Working Out at the Gym

*E*xercising at a gym can add variety to your workouts because you can use the diverse pieces of cardio and strength-training equipment as well as attend fitness classes. Enjoying your workouts is the key to staying consistent. If the gym, an aerobics class, or help from a personal trainer is your thing, stick with it. This chapter reviews what to look for when choosing a gym, which equipment to use, and how to pick the best teachers and trainers.

Heading for the Gym

Some people find the gym intimidating because of the huge machines and crowds of people, not to mention the sweaty hardbodies parading around for all to admire. Don't let that stop you from working out at a gym. You can get a great workout whether you're parading around in the newest look in spandex or sweats and a T-shirt. If you're bored working out at home and are motivated by the presence of others, then the gym just might be the answer.

The convenience factor

Location is the first consideration for most people when they're choosing a gym. If it's not convenient, chances are you won't go. First figure out what times you most enjoy working out, or when exercising fits into your schedule. If you like to work out at lunch or right after work, you may want a gym located near your office. On the other hand, if you like evening workouts or you're a weekend warrior, find a gym close to home.

Pick two or three gyms you're interested in joining and ask for a free day pass, or buy a week's visit. Trying a gym on for size helps you choose the one that's best for you. After all, you don't buy a car because you liked the commercial or a friend told you it was a good deal. You test drive it first, so you should give a gym a similar test run. Finding a gym that's convenient and fits your needs helps you keep your commitment to getting in shape.

A checklist for choosing a gym

As a consumer, you need to know what to look for in a fitness facility and what to ask before joining. Take a tour of the facilities you're interested in and consider the factors that are important to you before you sign up.

- How big is the facility?

    Some of the new super clubs can be overwhelming. Going into one is like entering a shopping mall. You can do and see so many things that you end up spending the day there. This isn't necessarily a bad thing, unless you have other obligations like going to work or picking your kids up from school. Smaller gyms can offer a more intimate workout environment and give you an opportunity to get to know the staff and members personally. On the down side, a small club may be limited in how many classes and types of equipment they offer.

- What are the fees? And does the gym offer any discounts or specials? Some gyms may give you a hard sell and try to sign you up for a membership that locks you in for a lifetime.

- What types of equipment does it have, is the equipment a quality name, is it in good shape, and does it fit your body properly? Unfortunately, many manufacturers design their equipment to fit an average size man. If that's not you, you may find it uncomfortable. Ask if the equipment can be adjusted enough to fit your body.

- How many pieces of equipment does the gym have? Is there a time limit on how long you can use each piece and do they have sign up sheets for them?

    Unavailability of the cardio machines like bikes and treadmills can cause rioting amongst members.

- Is the place clean?

    Check the bathrooms — they usually tell all.

- Does it have air conditioning or fans and good ventilation? Check it out at different times of the day. If the afternoon sun is shining brightly through the window, the temperature inside will increase.

✔ Is fresh water available?

✔ Does the gym offer its members towels if you forget to bring your own?

✔ Does it have showers, locker rooms to change in, and other bathroom amenities that are important to you?

✔ Does it offer other amenities you may desire, such as a juice or snack bar, massages, a sauna, a steam room, a Jacuzzi, personal trainers, nutritional/weight control counseling, audio and television hookups for the cardio room, or a pro shop?

✔ Does the club offer health screening for members, such as body fat testing, cardiovascular testing, and strength and flexibility testing?

✔ Does it limit the number of members it signs up, or does the gym try to pack in as many patrons as it can?

If you have to take a number to use the equipment, (like you do at the bakery), leave.

✔ What are the gym's hours, and when are the busiest times (after work, in the morning, and so on)?

✔ Does it offer childcare or kids' fitness classes?

✔ Does it offer adult fitness classes that appeal to you? How crowded are they, and at what times are they offered?

✔ Does the staff help you get started?

Watch out for gyms that sign you up and toss you into the lion's den without teaching you how to use any of the complex equipment, especially the new computerized pieces. I've seen a few people take flight off the treadmill. Taking a fall can be embarrassing, so figure out how to work each piece of equipment before they take you for a ride. Ask a staff member to give you a tour of the gym and show you how to use each piece of equipment, even if you don't think you'll ever touch it again. The next couple of times you come in, ask for help if you have forgotten how to work the machines. Most gyms help you design your own workout program and provide you with a fitness card to keep track of your workouts.

✔ Are the staff, trainers, and teachers qualified?

Do the trainers and teachers have any practical experience, certifications, or formal education? A few quality certifications to look for are: American College of Sports Medicine (ACSM), American Council on Exercise (ACE), Aerobics and Fitness Association of America (AFAA), National Academy of Sports Medicine (NASM), National Strength and Conditioning Association (NSCA), and the YMCA. Educational background may include degrees in physical education or exercise physiology.

Muscle-Conditioning Equipment

Resistance is what helps to develop your muscles. The two options listed here are machines designed to strengthen specific muscle groups and free weights (which can be used as a form of resistance in several ways to tone and build the muscles in your body).

Workout machines

You can do a lot of the exercises in this book at the gym by using their strength-training equipment. The manufacturers of weight-training machines, like Cybex and Nautilus, have created a piece of equipment that works every major muscle in your body. Take a list of your favorite exercises from this book and bring them to the gym with you. Chances are that if the gym has a good selection of equipment, you can find quite a few machines that replicate the same movement you are doing for the exercises in this book. If you don't find a piece that matches your selected exercise, ask one of the trainers to help you find a machine that exercises that muscle group. Most beginners enjoy using them because they reduce the risk of being injured or performing the exercise incorrectly. Machines, unlike free weights, have contained and attached weights that can't fall on you and are designed to place your body in correct form for performing the exercise. On the other hand, advanced exercisers can benefit from machines because such equipment allows you to increase the resistance of an exercise, pushing you to your limit, without needing the help of a spotter. (A spotter aids you in pushing beyond your limit by helping you lift a heavier amount of resistance.) Figure 19-1 shows you some samples of weight-training machines.

Free weights

Free weights and dumbbells are best used when you know what you're doing. Dropping a weight on your neighbor isn't going to make you a lot of friends. As you go through the exercises in this book, pay close attention to the tips on body form. Knowing how to perform an exercise correctly is your first step. All gyms have a few weight lifting "know-it-alls" (who really don't), so don't assume the guy on the bench next to you has a clue what he's doing. He may be using a technique he learned in junior high school from his best buddy. Your best bet is to educate yourself. If you're paying to use the gym's facilities, use the staff too. Let them show you how to use the equipment and how to perform the exercises. Figure 19-2 illustrates some typical free weights.

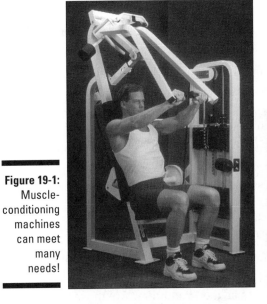

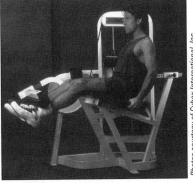

Photos courtesy of Cybex International, Inc.

Figure 19-1:
Muscle-conditioning machines can meet many needs!

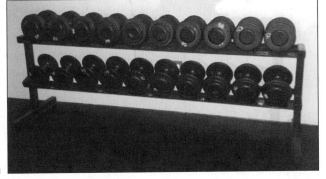

Figure 19-2:
Free weights are handy when you don't have machines.

Fitness Classes

Aerobic dance classes were rare until Judy Missett introduced us to Jazzercise back in the '70s. The craze began and leg warmers became a fashion statement. Before that we learned to exercise from one of the first instructors of fitness: Mr. Jack LaLane. He had us doing jumping jacks, push-ups, and leg lifts in front of our televisions. Fitness has come a long way, and the birth of group fitness classes has enabled millions of people to get in shape and enjoy the benefits of having a healthy body.

Although the aerobics industry has seen its share of trends and fashions, it's still going strong and is more diverse than ever before. If you plan to join a gym and attend its fitness classes, you may want to check out a few of the following things.

✔ Are the instructors certified, or do they have formal education or training in what they're teaching?

An A in a high school physical education class doesn't guarantee an instructor's ability to teach step aerobics.

✔ Does the aerobic room display safety signs and information on what to do in an emergency? (first aid, CPR, and so on)

✔ Does the instructor teach safety precautions in class and offer options for beginner exercisers?

✔ Does the amount of room in the facility allow students to move around without becoming too personal with the member next to them?

✔ Is the instructor or a staff member available before or after class to assist you and answer questions you may have pertaining to the class?

✔ Is the equipment used in class in good condition? Are the mats, floors, and mirrors clean?

✔ After you've given the class a try, did you enjoy it, and are you getting the results you expected from it?

Jazzercise started the craze in aerobic dance and now the industry is booming with fitness classes to enhance your heart, muscles, and mind. This brief list highlights some of the most traditional and trendiest classes.

High- and low-impact aerobics: A cardiovascular workout that combines high- and low-impact movements, such as kicking, jumping, and squatting, for a vigorous workout.

Step aerobics: An intense workout in which you elevate your heart rate by performing choreographed movements on an adjustable step.

Body sculpting/muscle conditioning: A fitness class dedicated to working your muscles using a variety of equipment like dumbbells, steps, bands, bars, and tubes.

Funk and Hip Hop: These low-impact aerobic classes get you dancing to funky music with choreographed club dance moves you commonly see on MTV rap videos.

Box aerobics: This class incorporates boxing techniques with aerobic dance to give you a great cardiovascular workout and help improve your balance, coordination, and agility.

Water aerobics: Doing aerobic dance moves in the water may be a bit slow-paced, but the water offers exercisers extra resistance and support. This class is great for pregnant women or people with joint problems.

Circuit: This class combines a variety of exercises, and participants rotate from one to the next at a quick pace.

Boot camp: A back-to-basics class that requires 100 percent of your effort. Classes typically incorporate sports drills, jump rope, sprinting, or stair running.

Spinning: This exercise class involves pedaling to music on a stationary bike. It's intense, but each bike has its own tension gauge so you can go as hard as you want or cut back and let your classmates pass you by.

Yoga: Yoga incorporates a true mind and body approach to fitness. This type of class challenges your body with stretching and strengthening positions and poses. Learning to balance your body while integrating deep breathing throughout the workout is the primary focus during this class. The concentration and focus needed to participate clear your mind and reduce your stress.

Tai Chi: [tie che] Slow motion movements, deep breathing, and concentration are emphasized in this ancient Chinese martial arts workout.

Pilates: [pill ot ees] Originally designed for dancers, these classes help improve your flexibility, strength, and posture. This workout is most commonly performed on a Pilates machine which has pulleys and cables. All movements are slow and controlled, and participants concentrate on deep breathing during each exercise.

Personal Trainers

In the past, personal trainers were considered a luxury for the rich and famous and were only found in health resorts and spas. That's not the case today. In fact, trainers are in high demand, and many consumers are choosing a one-to-one workout over group fitness classes. Trainers can be hired to get you in shape in a gym or in the privacy of your own home. Fees vary depending on where you live, the duration of your workout, and location of the actual training. Remember that you're paying not only for the trainer's knowledge and skills but also for the personal attention to you and only you.

A trainer's goals are to meet your specific fitness needs and help you accomplish *your* goals. The following checklist shows you what you should look for when working with a personal trainer.

- ✔ Is the trainer certified or does he or she have a related formal education? (See the list of certification organizations found at the end of the gym checklist in "A checklist for choosing a gym.")

- ✔ Are you the first client, or does the trainer have previous or current clients you can use as references?

- ✔ Did the trainer give you a fitness evaluation and work with you in designing a program that meets your needs?

- ✔ Does the trainer pay close attention to you and correct your techniques and form, or spend most of your session chatting about his or her last dinner date?

- ✔ Does the trainer introduce new exercises and equipment to you and educate you on how to perform or use them on your own?

- ✔ Does the trainer measure your progress and reassess your fitness needs and goals?

- ✔ Do you feel compatible with the trainer?

- ✔ Does he or she motivate you?

As a fitness instructor, for many years, I've enjoyed teaching my classes and getting feedback from my students at the gym. I've made a lot of friends and found some great workout partners, too. Although I do a great deal of my exercising at home, for me the gym adds variety to my workouts and my students continually motivate me to keep coming back for more.

Chapter 20

Special Workouts for Special Needs: Pregnancy, Seniors, and Kids

● ●

In This Chapter

▶ Building muscle for moms-to-be

▶ Maintaining senior stamina

▶ Setting a good example for your kids

● ●

Although the majority of this book addresses workouts for the general adult population, sometimes your body's physiology is so dramatically changed that your workouts must change as well. These dramatic changes are usually associated with age or a pregnancy. Despite your best efforts, you can't halt the aging process, and working out can become more difficult. A workout that stimulates a healthy young male football player may cripple an 80-year-old woman with osteoarthritis. The same workout probably doesn't suit an eight-year-old, either, due to a child's level of physical development. In addition, the change in body shape that accompanies a pregnancy can provide challenges in a standard workout.

The good news is, exercise can keep you feeling strong at any age, and during a pregnancy as well. As a fitness professional, I attempt to set up the proper program for each individual. Special topics in this chapter include workouts for expectant mothers and seniors, and the development of healthy habits for children.

Having a Baby . . . and Some Muscle

Congratulations! You're having a baby! You are probably so excited that you want to shout your news out to the world. You're glowing from head to toe and have a smile glued to your face. You're feeling good, looking good, and then it happens: Your body begins to change. Your breasts start to grow, and then your belly expands, so that soon it's announcing your arrival as you enter a room. Your ankles swell up, you feel your energy depleting rapidly, and you hope you don't end up with stretch marks.

Don't worry; there is hope. Exercising during pregnancy can enhance your energy level, self-esteem, and mood while your body goes through some of the discomforts of being pregnant. The secret to working out while pregnant is avoiding injury and harm to your baby. Although exercising throughout your pregnancy has many benefits, it's not always wise to start an exercise program if you don't already work out on a regular basis. In any case, check with your physician before beginning any workout program or continuing the one you are currently practicing.

Most research reports indicate that moderate exercise *does not* interfere with the growth of the fetus or harm the mother. In fact, many women who have gone through child birth give credit to their exercise programs for their ease of delivery and ability to get back into shape after delivery. Maintaining a healthy diet, exercising before pregnancy, and modifying your exercise during pregnancy can give you strength, stamina, and an outlet for stress. Continuing a workout program after childbirth helps you get back in shape and, more importantly, gives you the strength to pick up your child, carry the diaper bag, and the stroller, and the bottles, and the toys, and the . . .

Need I say more?

Your body's needs change during your pregnancy, so your workout program should be adjusted as you progress toward childbirth. Exercise classes specifically designed for pregnant women can teach you how to modify your current exercise regimen and provide you with safe alternative workouts for each stage of your pregnancy. Check with your local YMCA or gym for group or private exercise instruction for pregnant women.

My friend Mindy, the Super Mom

Mindy, a very close friend of mine, is an aerobics instructor who just turned forty and is also a mother of three. During one of our "girl talks" she explained to me how different each one of her pregnancies was and the amazing changes her body went through after each childbirth. Her in-depth description of what it was like to be pregnant and to give birth got a bit graphic and sounded a bit scary. You see, my "kids" have four legs and tend to be a little on the furry side. As Mindy saw the cheery smile on my face change to fear and concern, she reassured me that if a woman takes care of herself during and after her pregnancy, she has the ability to bounce back and be as good as new. She is living proof of the beauty of pregnancy. After each child, her body changed for the better. Mindy always makes fitness a part of her lifestyle before, during, and after her pregnancies. Her lifelong commitment to her health and well-being has benefited her, and she has become a wonderful role model for her three kids. She's one great mom!

A general list of do's and don'ts

A thorough medical exam by your obstetrician/gynecologist can ascertain any pregnancy-related complications you may have and what modifications you may need to make in your lifestyle. After your doctor has given you the go ahead to begin a prenatal exercise program, you should abide by some general safety rules, shown in these lists of do's and don'ts.

Do's

- ✔ **Do warm up** before you work out, and cool down afterward. (See Chapter 4 for hints on each of these activities.)

- ✔ **Do be cautious not to overheat** during your workout, especially in your first trimester.

- ✔ **Do keep yourself hydrated** by drinking plenty of water.

- ✔ **Do modify your exercise exertion level** and maintain a safe target heart rate range. In general, heart rate should not exceed 140 beats per minute.

- ✔ **Do increase your flexibility** by moving through your exercises slowly, and don't overextend your stretches.

- ✔ **Do perform low intensity cardiovascular exercises** such as walking and swimming.

- ✔ **Do check into fitness classes** designed specifically for pregnant women.

- ✔ **Do enjoy saying, "I don't have a beer belly — I'm pregnant,"** for the next nine months.

Don'ts

- ✔ **Don't exercise in extremely hot or humid weather.**

- ✔ **Don't exercise too intensely** or for prolonged periods of time. This may impair fetal blood flow.

- ✔ **Don't strain yourself while lifting weights.** Have someone spot you while you weight train.

- ✔ **Don't try to lift a lot of weight.** Use lighter weights and perform more repetitions.

- ✔ **Don't continue an exercise if you feel pain** or discomfort.

- ✔ **Don't hold your breath** at any point during your exercise.

- ✔ **Don't exercise on your back after the first trimester.** This places undue mechanical stress on the abdominal wall and also decreases circulation to the fetus.

Following pregnancy workout guidelines

When you work out, follow these general guidelines from the American College of Obstetricians and Gynecologists for a safe and healthy exercise program. These guidelines originate from the pamphlet *Exercise During Pregnancy* (Patient Education Pamphlet No. AP119), Washington, DC, © ACOG, May 1998.

- ✔ After 20 weeks of pregnancy, avoid doing any exercise on your back.
- ✔ Avoid brisk exercise in hot, humid weather or when you're sick with a fever.
- ✔ Wear comfortable clothing that helps you to remain cool.
- ✔ Wear a bra that fits well and gives lots of support to help protect your breasts.
- ✔ Drink plenty of water to help keep you from overheating and dehydrating.
- ✔ Make sure you consume the extra 300 calories a day you need during pregnancy.

While you exercise, pay attention to your body. Don't exercise to the point where you're exhausted. Be aware of the warning signs that you may be exercising too strenuously. If you notice any of the following symptoms, stop exercising and call your doctor.

- ✔ Pain
- ✔ Vaginal bleeding
- ✔ Dizziness or feeling faint
- ✔ Increased shortness of breath
- ✔ Rapid heartbeat
- ✔ Difficulty walking
- ✔ Uterine contractions and chest pain
- ✔ Fluid leaking from the vagina

Changes in Your Body

Pregnancy causes many changes in your body. Some of these changes can affect your ability to exercise.

- ✔ **Joints:** The hormones produced during pregnancy cause the ligaments that support your joints to become relaxed. This makes the joints more mobile and more at risk for injury. Avoid jerky, bouncy, or high-impact motions that can increase your risk of injury.

✔ **Balance:** Remember that during pregnancy you are carrying extra pounds — as many as 20 to 30 pounds at the end of pregnancy. The extra weight in the front of your body shifts your center of gravity and places stress on joints and muscles, especially those in the pelvis and lower back. This can make you less stable, cause back pain, and make you more likely to lose your balance and fall, especially in later pregnancy.

✔ **Heart rate:** The extra weight you're carrying makes your body work harder than it did before you were pregnant. Exercise increases the flow of oxygen and blood to the muscles being worked, and away from other parts of your body, so it's important not to overdo it.

Try to exercise moderately so that you don't get tired quickly. If you are unable to talk normally while exercising, your activity is too strenuous.

Planning a Pregnancy Workout

This pregnancy exercise routine is a general workout for moms-to-be. Remember that all exercises have to be varied depending on the stage of your pregnancy and your level of fitness. Before attempting the exercises below or starting any new form of exercise program, please check with your physician. Your needs may be different from another woman's, and your pregnancy may have different effects on your body. Your doctor can assess which forms of exercise are best for you at this point in your pregnancy, and what the frequency and duration of your workouts should be. Table 20-1 gives you some general guidelines for warming up, cardiovascular exercise, and muscle conditioning. This exercise prescription varies depending on which trimester you are in as well as your current level of health. The table is followed by some recommended muscle exercises.

Pelvic tilt

The pelvic tilt, shown in Figure 20-1, strengthens your back and abdominals — two very important areas during pregnancy. A strong torso can provide you with the support you need as your body continues to change and grow.

1. **Place your hands and knees on the floor and keep your neck and back parallel with the floor. Don't allow the weight of your belly to cause an excessive arch in your back.**

2. **Lightly contract your abdominals and arch your back upward. Allow your head to drop by pulling your chin in to your chest.**

3. **Release and repeat.**

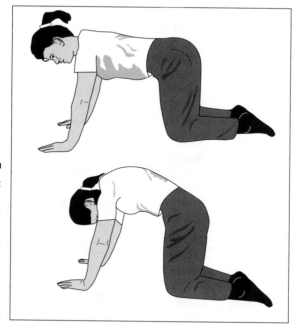

Figure 20-1:
The pelvic tilt can strengthen your back and abs for ease in everyday tasks.

Table 20-1	General Guidelines for Pregnant Exercisers	
	How Long?	*What To Do:*
Warming up	5 minutes	Walk or march in place while swinging your arms forward and back.
Cardiovascular	15 minutes (or longer if you've exercised prior to pregnancy)	Light intensity: walking, biking, swimming, water aerobics, or a prenatal aerobic class.
	5 minutes (cool down)	Do the same activity at a much lower intensity.
Muscle-conditioning exercises	15 to 20 minutes twice a week is a safe guideline to follow, but check with your doctor to see what is best recommended for your body	Resistance training exercises using relatively light weights (2 to 8 pounds, or 0.9 to 3.6 kg) and keeping the intensity light, unless otherwise specified. Attempt 8 to 10 repetitions broken into 1 or more sets, depending on your physical condition and ability.

Bicep curl

Strengthening your bicep muscles with the move shown in Figure 20-2 helps prepare you to carry around your new bundle of joy. Remember, you'll soon be carrying a diaper bag along with your baby, so you need to increase your strength.

1. **Sit in a chair and place your feet on the floor.**

   Keep your back straight and maintain good posture.

2. **Place a dumbbell in each hand and hold them to the side of each thigh, with your palms up.**

3. **Contract your biceps by pulling the weights toward your shoulders. Release and repeat.**

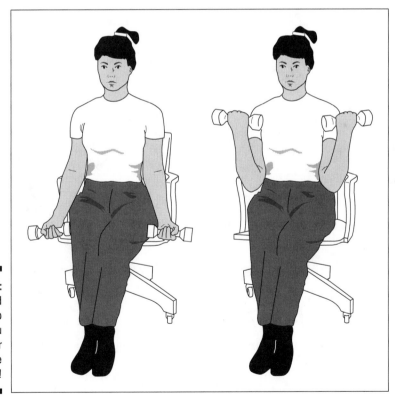

Figure 20-2:
A good shape-up before you carry your new little one!

Tricep counter dip

The exercise in Figure 20-3 may be difficult if you haven't exercised your tricep muscles prior to your pregnancy. Pregnancy causes difficulty in finding your center of balance, so you may choose to modify this exercise by bending your elbows only slightly or by having a partner assist you.

1. **Face away from a desk or counter and place your hands behind you on the countertop with your palms down and fingers facing forward.**

2. **Bring your feet slightly out in front of you, but be aware of your balance.**

3. **Slowly lower yourself by flexing your elbows and bending your knees.**

4. **Keep the majority of your weight in your upper arms and push yourself back up to the starting position. Repeat the exercise.**

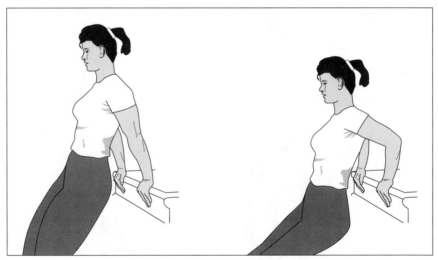

Figure 20-3:
Watch your balance when performing the tricep counter dip.

Wall push-ups

Push-ups are a great exercise to develop strength in your chest, shoulders, biceps, and triceps. You can still perform this popular exercise by reducing the degree of difficulty. When using a wall for your push-ups, shown in Figure 20-4, make sure you tighten your abdominal muscles to support your torso, and avoid allowing the weight of your belly to pull you forward.

1. **Stand facing a wall and place your hands against the wall at about shoulder level, slightly wider apart than your body.**

2. Take a step or two away from the wall so that your body is at a slight angle to the wall.

3. Lower yourself toward the wall, letting your elbows flex.

4. Push yourself back to the starting position and repeat the exercise.

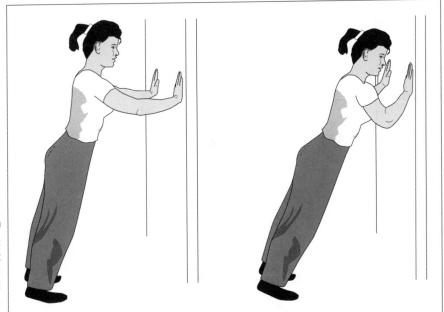

Figure 20-4:
A new twist on the traditional push-up.

Side arm raises

Exercising your shoulder muscles with the move shown in Figure 20-5 gives you greater strength for many of your daily activities during and after your pregnancy.

1. **Stand with your feet shoulder-width apart and place a dumbbell in each hand.**

2. **Keeping only a slight bend in your elbow and your palms down, lift both hands out to your sides until they reach your shoulder level.**

3. **Maintain good posture and don't sway forward as you lift. (You can do this exercise in a chair for more back support.)**

4. **Lower your arms and repeat the exercise.**

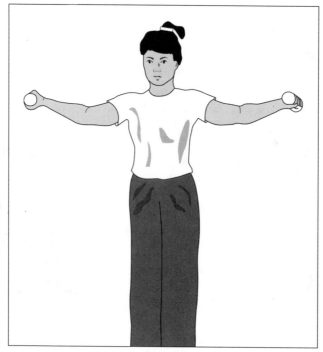

Arm and leg reach

I call the exercise in Figure 20-6 the arm and leg reach, but it actually works your back muscles. This one looks like swimming on dry land. You don't have water to keep you afloat, so be careful of your balance while performing this exercise.

1. **Place your hands and knees on the floor and a pillow under your knees for comfort.**

2. **Keep your neck and back parallel with the floor and don't allow your belly to create an excessive arch in your back.**

3. **Simultaneously lift one arm and the opposing leg up so that they become parallel with your torso.**

4. **Alternate each arm lift with an opposing leg lift.**

   If this exercise is uncomfortable or causes you to lose your balance, you can break up the exercise by first alternating the arm lifts only and then alternating the leg lifts while keeping both hands on the floor.

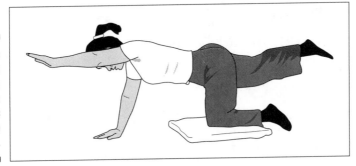

Figure 20-6:
The arm and leg reach requires some balance.

Side leg lift

You'll probably feel comfortable in the position shown in Figure 20-7. Your legs carry extra weight throughout your pregnancy, so you'll want to build muscle in your legs and buns.

1. **Lie on your side and prop yourself up on your elbow, or relax your torso and head on the floor. You may want to place a towel under your hip for comfort.**

2. **Place your top arm in front of you with your hand on the floor for support and balance. Lift your top leg up, squeezing your outer thigh and buns.**

3. **Release and repeat, using your other leg.**

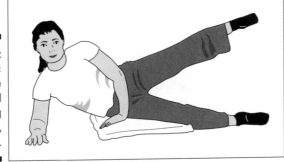

Figure 20- 7:
This classic exercise works well during pregnancy, too.

Side adductor lift

Toned inner thighs tend to be a popular desire of many women before and after they have children. Keep your thighs in shape by continuing to exercise them throughout your pregnancy, using the move shown in Figure 20-8.

1. **Lie on your side and prop yourself up on your elbow, or relax your torso and head on the floor. You may want to place a towel under your hip for comfort.**

2. **Place your top arm in front of you with your hand on the floor for support and balance.**

3. **Place your top leg behind your lower leg with your knee bent and foot on the floor.**

4. **Lift your lower leg toward the ceiling, keeping your foot flexed. Release and repeat, using your other leg.**

Figure 20-8: You can maintain strong thighs before and after you have your baby.

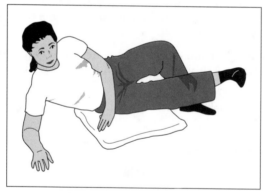

Hip extension lift

A pillow can add a little comfort to the exercise shown in Figure 20-9, which works your buns and the back of your thighs. Concentrate on squeezing your buns as you lift your leg up.

1. **Place your knees and elbows on the floor. Keep your neck and torso in a straight line with your head, but angled toward the floor.**

2. **Alternate lifting each leg up and out so that it becomes level with your torso. Don't arch your back to lift your leg higher.**

3. **Release and repeat, using your other leg.**

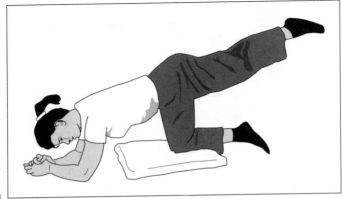

Figure 20-9:
Keep your
legs strong
to carry you
through
each
trimester.

Exercising Your Seniority

When you ask children their ages, they are always eager to tell you how old they will soon be. You may hear them say, "I'll be nine this summer," which may be six months away. When you ask adults their ages, you may hear, "I just turned 35 six months ago." You usually don't hear, "I'll be 36 in six months." At some point in the aging process, many people lose their eagerness to grow older and develop a desire to be younger than they are.

What does your age really mean? When do you consider yourself a senior? Do you look as old as you feel or do you feel as old as you look? You may answer these subjective questions any way you like, but the fact remains that you do age and your body does grow old. If you make a commitment to maintain your health and fitness, you can continue to feel and look good.

Growing old is a normal biological process. Today's technology and medicine make it possible for us to live longer and healthier lives. Unfortunately, even if you are able to live 90 or more years, your body still deteriorates as those years pass by. Around the 40-year mark you may notice your body doesn't move as fast, lose weight as quickly, or recover as readily as it did in the past. I'm reaching that landmark age myself and realizing that no matter how much I fight it, my body is still going to age. The fortunate — or for some people, unfortunate — thing is that what you do to your body throughout your life span determines just how fast your level of health and fitness will decline. Choosing to make exercise a part of your lifestyle can enhance and strengthen your body and mind, slowing down the aging process.

Unfortunately, in our society, aging is somewhat frowned upon (no pun intended). You usually don't hear people saying, "Wow! Look at that attractive elderly person." And you probably don't walk around saying, "Yahoo! I'm getting old," unless, of course, you're about to turn 21. In that case, you don't need to read this section.

You're more likely to hear comments like, "She's over the hill," "He's all washed up," or "Your hair's such a nice color of blue." Get my drift? The fact is, your body is built to evolve on a cycle. Once you reach the peak of that cycle you begin to slow down, both looking physically different and responding differently. For example, if you run 10 miles a day at age 25, you are in top physical shape. To maintain this level of ability and physical condition at age 50, you would probably have to work twice as hard as you did when you were 25. Personally, I choose to graciously decline. Aside from the fact that I didn't like running even when I was 25, I realize that I can enjoy the changes my body is going through by providing it with the right amount of exercise for my age and ability.

Benefiting from staying fit

To maintain your quality of life and extend your longevity, it is important to eat right and to exercise. Evidence indicates many positive factors of exercising for the elderly. Benefits include:

- Cardiovascular and pulmonary (heart function) improvement
- Disease and arthritis prevention
- Improved coordination and balance
- Increases in and/or maintenance of bone density (prevention of osteoporosis)
- Increased endurance, strength, and stamina through resistance training exercises
- Increased flexibility
- Prevention of muscle and nerve deterioration
- Enhances metabolic fitness (your ability to burn calories and fat)
- Prevention of unnecessary injury due to falls or common accidents
- Slowing down of the aging process and improved quality of life

Workouts for seniors

The most recommended workout routine for seniors is a combination of resistance training exercises with bands or light weights, and cardiovascular exercise. If you are beginning an exercise program, first consult with your physician, then look for a program designed for senior fitness. The key is to begin at a comfortable pace and increase the intensity of your program gradually. The following workout is a basic program designed specifically for seniors. Your end goal is to have fun and improve the quality of your life by staying fit.

Cardiovascular exercise

Increasing your heart rate won't be as easy as it was when you were in your twenties, but it's just as important. Cardiovascular fitness is a vital element in keeping a healthy heart and overall positive well-being.

- Always warm up before beginning your exercise and cool down once you have finished (see Chapter 4 for tips).

- Perform 20 minutes of exercise, 3 to 5 times per week.

- Keep your exercise at a low to moderate intensity, approximately 55 percent to 65 percent of your maximum heart rate (see Chapter 10 for heart rate charts).

- Choose low-impact exercises like walking, swimming, bicycling, using a stair climber, low-impact dance aerobics, and chair aerobics.

Muscle-conditioning exercise

Overall loss of muscles cells can be prevented by doing resistance training exercises. As you can see from the variety of benefits listed in the previous section, maintaining a fit body can slow down the aging process and enhance your overall lifestyle.

You can use the following guidelines when doing the rubber band workout that follows in this chapter.

- Perform 20 to 30 minutes of resistance training exercises, a minimum of 2 times per week.

- Perform one exercise for each muscle group with at least one set of approximately 8 to 10 repetitions. (Example: You exercise your buns by doing one set of 10 repetitions of chair squats.)

- Choose 8 to 10 different muscle groups to exercise for each workout.

✔ Use relatively light weights or bands, and try to gradually increase the number of repetitions of each exercise you do to increase your muscle endurance.

 ✔ Flexibility is important at every age and can help prevent injury, so aim for a goal of stretching a little bit every day. Try to spend 30 minutes stretching after your workout to keep yourself limber.

The Senior Band workout that follows shows you 10 different exercises that can condition your whole body. You can follow this program easily by doing each exercise listed a total of 8 to 10 times. This means you do 1 set of 8 to 10 repetitions (reps) for all ten exercises. If you can do more sets, more power to you!

The Senior Band Workout

You may notice, if you scan through the entire book, that I love to work out with exercise bands. I find that people of all ages enjoy and benefit from this form of resistance. Due to the aging process, older adults tend to be prone to injury and should avoid intense or excessive amounts of exercise. Working out with heavy weights or doing fast, bouncing aerobic moves may feel awkward and difficult, so I like to recommend using a rubber band.

Seated front-thigh extension

Don't kick anyone — just extend your knee and start working your quadriceps (the front of your thigh). The move in Figure 20-10 can give you added strength when you walk or even when you just get up and out of a chair.

1. **Sit in a chair and place the band around your ankles.**

2. **Begin with both feet placed on the floor and then extend one leg up to knee level.**

3. **Slowly lower your foot back to the starting position and repeat using your other leg.**

Seated outer-thigh press out

Have a seat and exercise your outer thighs with the exercise shown in Figure 20-11. Be careful not to let your legs snap back in; keep the band in control as you bring your legs back to the center of your body.

1. **Sit in a chair and place the band around your ankles.**

2. Hold on to the sides of the chair for support.

3. Slowly open your legs up by squeezing your outer thighs. Slowly release your legs to their starting position and repeat.

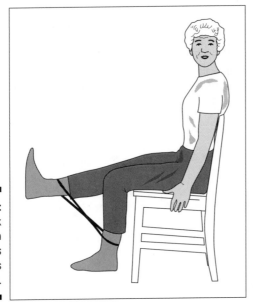

Figure 20-10: Don't kick anyone in the pants with this exercise.

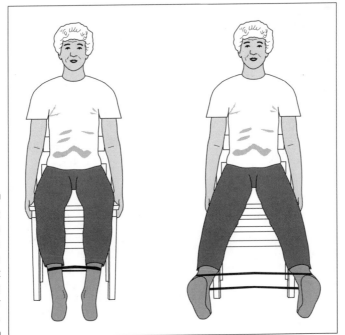

Figure 20-11: It's easy to get a tough thigh workout while sitting in your chair.

Seated inner-thigh leg lift

You can actually get a two-for-one deal with the exercise in Figure 20-12. If you tighten your abdominals as you lift your leg, you can exercise your inner thighs and make your abs work too.

1. **Sit in a chair and place the band around your ankles.**

2. **Hold on to the chair for support.**

3. **Bring one leg out and across your body, squeezing the inner thigh muscles. Your heel should be positioned toward the ceiling.**

4. **Repeat using your other leg.**

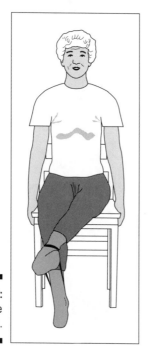

Figure 20-12:
Two for the
lift of one.

Standing back-thigh curl

It is natural to want to arch your back while doing the hamstring curl in Figure 20-13, but doing so isn't safe. If you contract your abs, you help support your lower back and prevent excessive arching as you lift your foot to your buns.

1. **Place the band around your ankles and balance yourself using the back of a chair as support. Keep your knees slightly bent and don't arch your back extensively.**

2. **Flex one foot and lift your heel toward your buns.**

3. **Slowly release the tension by bringing your foot down. Repeat using your other leg.**

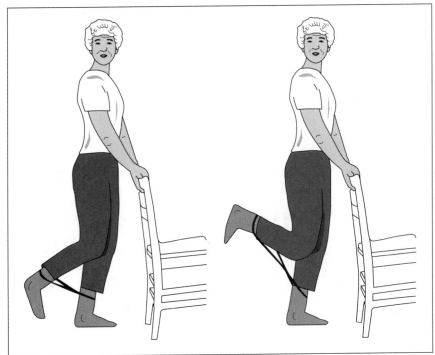

Figure 20-13: Focus on exercising the back of your thigh without excessively arching your back.

Chest presses

Keep your pectoral muscles strong with the chest press shown in Figure 20-14. Have a seat in a chair for support, but remember to keep your back straight (no slouching) and focus on your chest muscles.

1. **Grip the inside of the band with your palms facing out.**

2. **Lift your arms to chest level, keeping your wrists in line with your forearms. Tighten your abdominals and maintain good posture throughout the exercise.**

3. **Keeping your elbows slightly bent, press your arms out as far as you can.**

4. **Slowly release your arms and repeat the exercise.**

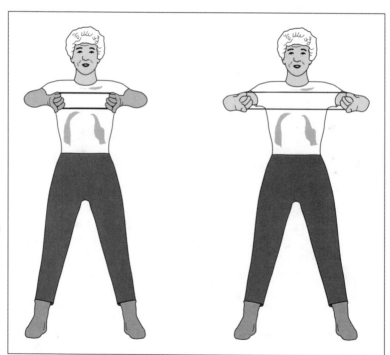

Figure 20-14:
Chest presses can help maintain good posture.

Seated upright row

You need to make sure your band is placed securely under your feet before you begin to exercise your shoulders with the move in Figure 20-15.

1. Sit in a chair and place the band under the arches of both your feet. Make sure the band is secure by stepping on it — you don't want it to pop out from under your feet.

2. Hold on to the opposite end of the band with both hands, keeping your elbows bent and palms facing in.

3. Pull the band toward your chest and resist back down. Repeat the exercise.

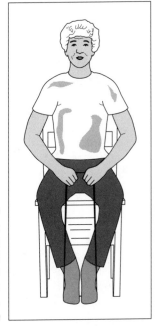

Figure 20-15:
Position the band securely for this exercise.

Upper-back pullback

The exercise in Figure 20-16 is a key to maintaining good posture. Remember to concentrate on tightening the muscles of your upper back as you pull the rubber band across your chest.

1. Hold the band with each fist and raise your fists to shoulder level so that your elbows are raised up and out. Keep your abdominals tight and maintain good posture.

2. Pull your elbows toward your back by contracting your upper-back muscles.

3. Release the band slowly and repeat the exercise.

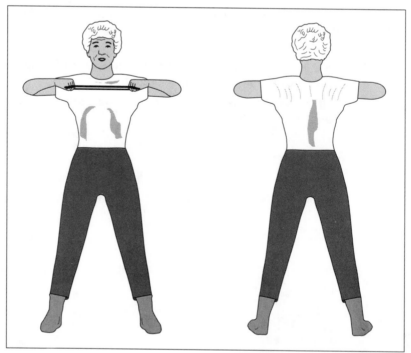

Figure 20-16:
This move
helps
maintain
good
posture.

Upper-arm press back

The exercise shown in Figure 20-17 helps you get out of bed a little easier in the morning by working your tricpes. Just press the band back behind you, maintaining control as you release it.

1. **Grab the end of the band with one hand and press it against your waist on the opposite side.**

2. **Place your other hand inside the band, palm facing out. Hold it behind your back, bending your elbow.**

3. **Extend the elbow of the arm behind you by pressing your palm backward. Don't flex your torso forward as you extend your arm.**

4. **Slowly release your hand and repeat the exercise, using your other arm.**

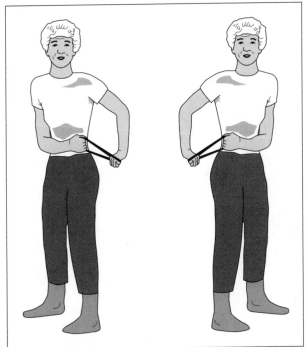

Figure 20-17:
This move
strengthens
your triceps
and your
pushing
ability.

Seated arm curl

Good bicep muscles are a bonus in many of your daily activities, and the exercise in Figure 20-18 helps you maintain them. Lift the band as high as you can and release it in a slow, controlled motion.

1. **Sit in a chair and place the band under the arch of one foot.**

2. **Hold the other end of the band with your hand of the same side as the foot.**

3. **With your palm facing up, pull the band toward your chest by contracting your bicep muscle (upper arm). Keep your elbow close to your body and your foot secure on the floor.**

4. **Slowly lower the band and repeat the exercise using your other arm.**

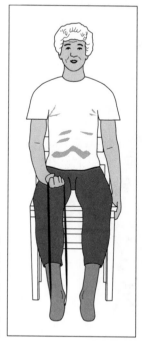

Figure 20-18:
On your
way to
better
biceps.

Upper-back strengthener

You can do the exercise in Figure 20-19 while lying comfortably on the floor. Make your movements small, and focus on your back muscles.

1. **Lie on the floor face down and place a towel under your hips for comfort.**

2. **Hold the band with both fists, palms facing inward, and extend your arms above your head. You don't need to pull the band excessively, but keep it taut by slightly pulling either end.**

3. **Relax your body, then lift both arms off the floor as high as you can without lifting your chest off the ground.**

4. **Hold that position for 2 counts, release your arms, and repeat the exercise.**

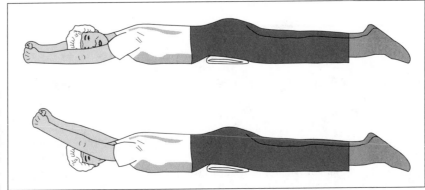

Figure 20-19:
The essential back strengthener.

Abdominal curl

Strong backs are complemented with strong abs, so don't forget to exercise the front of your torso. Remember to keep your chin off your chest as you lift your shoulders off the ground (see Figure 20-20). Crossing your ankles may add a bit of comfort to your curls.

1. **Lie on your back and place your hands behind your head.**

2. **Cross your ankles and pull your knees in slightly toward your chest.**

3. **Keeping your chin off your chest, lift your shoulders and chest toward the ceiling.**

4. **Hold the contraction for a second or two, then slowly lower yourself back to the starting position and repeat the exercise.**

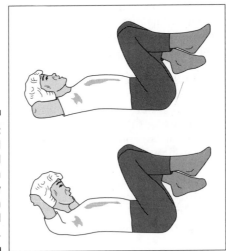

Figure 20-20:
Keep good abdominal strength and stability with abdominal curls.

TAMILEE SAYS

Fitness as a lifestyle

As a fitness educator, I hope to experience teaching people of all fitness levels and all age groups. One day I was asked to speak on the topic of aging at a senior citizen health conference. I was thrilled to be asked, but as time went by, I realized I wasn't sure what to write my lecture about. What should I say to an audience of individuals 20 or more years older than I? As my turn to speak approached, I allowed the words to come from my intuition and knowledge of fitness. Though I can't recall the exact words I spoke, my thoughts were something like this: "The minute we are conceived we begin growing. The second we are born we begin aging, and we don't stop until our lives end. Our choice of lifestyles and how we care for our minds and bodies during these years has an effect on the rest of our lives. Our bodies become very important to us when we are in our teens, and during that time we are mostly concerned with what we look like rather than how we feel. We tend to take our bodies and our health for granted in our younger years, assuming we'll always be able to bounce back no matter what we do. As we approach midlife, our thoughts begin to focus more on our internal health instead of just how we look on the outside. Aging can be a beautiful thing if we are able to focus on taking care of ourselves from the inside out. With each year, do your best to keep your body and your mind moving."

Kids in Motion

When I was a kid, few people had computers, computer games, or a TV set in their rooms. (No, it wasn't that long ago, and yes, we did have color TV back then.) We did our homework as soon as we got home from school and then went out to play until we had to come in for dinner. The TV was never turned on until after we cleaned the dinner dishes. Back then, little was said about kids having weight problems. This may be because most kids received enough exercise. We were out playing, not sitting in front of the TV or computer every day for several hours.

I'm not knocking technology, but it's important to maintain a balance between enhancing our minds and enhancing our health. Unfortunately, current statistics show that 20 percent of the nation's children from the ages of 5 to 17 are considered obese. To make things worse, these children have a greater chance of growing up to be obese adults. This problem usually begins at home, and if you're a parent, it's your responsibility to set an example of a healthy lifestyle.

Try combining your workouts with your children's. Make your activities a family event — go for a bike ride or in-line skate together. These activities are fun for the whole family and give you quality time with your children.

Getting kids interested and involved in exercise and sports activities that they find enjoyable is the easiest way to keep them in shape and help them establish a lifetime of fitness interests.

Unlike many adults who see the benefits of fitness as "tight buns and abs," kids view fitness and sports activities as a way to socialize, be competitive, and have fun.

Kids can benefit from exercise in many ways:

- Exercise can help in the prevention of heart disease.
- Maintaining an active lifestyle can reduce and control high blood pressure.
- Being active and eating a healthy diet can help kids maintain a healthy weight and avoid childhood obesity. Unfit, obese children tend to become unfit, obese adults.
- Exercise helps kids develop motor skills, improve their agility, and increase their flexibility and balance.
- Sports and fitness activities can increase a child's confidence and self-esteem.
- Making fitness a part of a child's early years helps develop and instill a lifetime of healthy habits.

Workout guidelines for kids

Aside from being a good role model for your kids, you can help them develop healthy habits by knowing the basic guidelines for kids' fitness. For many children, play time is an adequate amount of physical activity to keep them fit. If your child is interested in a fitness program, I advise that you check with his or her physician for specific guidelines and follow the general recommendations below.

Intensity

Just as adults should, your kids should begin an exercise program slowly and gradually increase the intensity.

Duration

Workouts that last 20 to 30 minutes at a time is a good goal, but start kids out with less time and gradually increase the duration. This guideline may depend on the activity or sport. You know if the duration is too long if kids get bored and don't want to play your "exercise game" anymore.

Frequency

Two to three times per week is an adequate number of days for a kids' fitness program. Make sure they get a day of rest in between each workout.

Children go through developmental stages as they age and their bodies require different needs than those of adults. Take the following precautions if your kids want to work out:

- Children should avoid heavy weight lifting because of the growth of their bones and development of their joints.
- Beware when exercising in extremely hot or cold weather. The body temperature regulation of children is immature.
- Kids' heart rates and breathing patterns are more variable than adults' and should not be compared to charts designed for adults.

Where to find special programs

Check your local gym to see if they offer kids' fitness programs. Another alternative is your neighborhood YMCA, which not only offers fitness programs, but usually offers sports teams or camps where instructors teach kids proper form and how to play sports. Team activities also give kids a chance to interact with other kids.

Ten of the most fun activities for kids . . .

. . . recommended by my best friends under the age of 16.

- Bike riding
- Dancing
- In-line skating
- Jumping rope
- Playing games like dodgeball, tag, and kickball
- Playing hopscotch
- Playing sports like soccer, baseball, and basketball
- Skateboarding
- Swimming and playing pool games like Marco Polo
- Tumbling and jumping on a trampoline

Part VI
The Part of Tens

The 5th Wave   By Rich Tennant

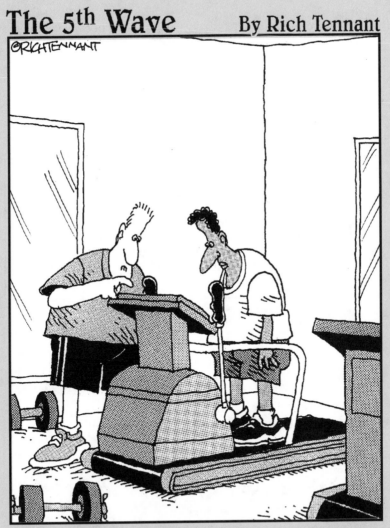

"This readout shows your heart rate, blood pressure, bone density, skin hydration, plaque buildup, liver function, and expected lifetime!"

In this part . . .

I list my ten favorite videos, which I happen to be the creator of, plus my ten favorite fitness books, and favorite exercises. These chapters provide you with the resources to keep you motivated and keep you moving.

Chapter 21

My Ten Favorite Exercises and Why You Should Do Them

▶ My top ten moves

▶ *Why* they're my top ten moves

*Y*ou probably have some favorite exercises, but this chapter shows you my top ten. You can bet that all of them are a part of my weekly workouts. Why do I keep exercising? First of all, it keeps me employed — but more importantly, I enjoy it and I wouldn't give up the benefits of having a healthy body for anything.

Favorite Exercises

I've performed and created a lot of different exercises for my classes and videos, but a select number always seem to be "must-haves" for each workout. The following ten exercises are my (and my students') favorites. Each has a universal appeal to both men and women. (Well, with the exception of the plié; for some reason, most men don't enjoy working their inner thighs by spreading their feet and performing squats.) The real appeal of these exercises doesn't necessarily come from the pleasure of performing them, but rather from the rewards after you repeatedly do them.

Lunges

This exercise is a sure bet. I do it because it gets me results. You can do lunges a variety of ways, but they all come down to the same thing — bun blasting.

Chapter 15 has all the information you need on lunges.

Squats

The squat has been called the grandfather of all exercises — probably because it's been around a long time and still does the job. The other great thing about squats is that they exercise several muscle groups: your quads, buns, and hamstrings.

See Chapter 13 for details on squats.

Tricep dips

Dips are an effective and easy way to exercise your triceps. Well, they may not necessarily be easy to do, but you can do them just about anywhere. The convenience factor of this exercise is even greater because you use your own body weight as resistance — so you don't even need any equipment.

See Chapter 10 for details on tricep dips.

Push-ups

You don't have to be in the armed forces to get all the great benefits of doing push-ups. This is always one of the exercises I take on the road with me. I can exercise my chest and arms in one exercise, and as long as I have a floor, I'm good to go.

Chapter 10 tells you what you want to know about push-ups.

Abdominal crunches

This basic ab exercise puts it all together in one tight crunch. I can get a great abdominal workout by focusing on tightening the lower and upper portion of my abdominals at the same time.

See Chapter 12 for the abdominal crunch exercise.

Side leg lifts with the band

How can you go wrong with an exercise that is so easy? I can work my thighs when I'm cooking in the kitchen by just placing my SPRI rubber band around my ankles and doing leg lifts. By waddling around my kitchen with the rubber band on, I can keep working out even when I'm baking a cake.

Chapter 16 has the lowdown on the side leg lifts with the band.

Pliés

In this exercise, I get to pretend I'm as graceful as a ballerina. If any of you have seen my ballet moves, you'll know why I *pretend*. Fortunately, you don't need to be graceful to get a great inner-thigh workout from doing pliés, and you don't need a ballet bar to do them.

Look for plié information in Chapter 14.

Double upper-arm curls with the Exercise Bar

I love my Exercise Bar. It's like a barbell, but I don't have to deal with putting on and taking off the weights in order to change the difficulty of the exercise. All I have to do is turn the bar to tighten the tube and bam! — the same exercise becomes more challenging. My biceps get a great workout with these basic bar curls.

See Chapter 17 for all the details on the double upper-arm curls with the Exercise Bar.

Overhead shoulder press

I'm not sure why I really like this shoulder exercise . . . maybe because it makes me feel like Atlas when I lift heavy objects over my head. The bottom line is that the shoulder press gets the results I'm looking for.

Check out Chapter 11 for what you need to know about the overhead shoulder press.

Upright shoulder rows with the Exercise Bar

Upright shoulder rows seem to be so much easier for me to do with the Exercise Bar. The movements are smooth, and I can feel my shoulder muscles working every step of the way.

See Chapter 17 for details on upright shoulder rows with the Exercise Bar.

Jumping on beds

My editor told me he couldn't do this exercise because his mom told him not to. Well, I'm sure my mom told me, too, so let's not show her this page.

Chapter 17 provides information for jumping on beds.

Chapter 22
Tamilee's Top Ten Workout Videos

After starring in a total of 52 videos, 22 of them part of the "Buns of Steel" collection, I have faith that one or more of the videos in this chapter can help you achieve your fitness goals. The following list gives you my top ten favorites. This chapter may seem a bit self-promoting, but I've highlighted ten of my best videos for you because they're consistent with the ideas and workouts included in this book. I even included some excerpts from letters I received from dedicated video fans to give you a little extra motivation.

Working out with a consistent program is important, but any workout is better than no workout, and variety can spice up your exercise routine. Keeping that in mind, I highlight other excellent videos at the end of the chapter.

Classic Buns of Steel

This is my first Buns of Steel video. If you ever work out to this video, you'll notice I seem to have a lisp — but actually, the video production had sound problems that caused a "sssp" at the end of all my words. Maybe the sound problem happened for a reason, because now you can laugh at me through your workout instead of concentrating on how tired you are doing all the squats and lunges. This Buns video takes you through a complete workout, focusing on firming up your buns, thighs, and upper legs. It was voted *Best Lower Body Exercise Video* in 1992 by *Self* magazine.

Testimonial: About a year and a half ago, I looked in the mirror and made myself a promise to get healthy! After exercising to your videos (and eating a healthy diet like you stress) on a regular basis, I am down 35 pounds! I'm so grateful, Tamilee, for the encouraging workouts you've designed. You're always smiling and saying, "C'mon, I know you can do it!" And I did.

Abs of Steel

This is my first video to make the Billboard Top Ten charts. In fact, Abs of Steel hit the number one spot and remained there for five years straight. I have received thousands of letters of appreciation regarding this tape from both men and women. This workout video consists of three 10-minute abdominal programs concentrated on toning and tightening your abs.

Classic Abs of Steel

After the success of the first abs video, I had to come up with more advanced exercises for the men and women who are die-hard ab maniacs. This Abs of Steel video consists of two 15-minute workouts that can get you on your way to washboard abs and create definition around your waist. During this program you do intervals of push-ups. Why? Because push-ups not only work your chest, shoulders, and arms, they also make you contract your abdominals. As you elevate your body, to perform the exercise properly you must contract your abdominal muscles, which support the erector spinea muscle in your back. Toning up your abdominals not only helps you shed the love handles — it also protects and gives support to your back.

Legs of Steel

Legs of Steel is all about your thighs, quads, hamstrings, and calves. And, of course, I wouldn't leave out your buns. The idea was actually inspired by Buns of Steel fans begging for more leg exercises. These exercises are designed to tone and firm up your body from the hips on down.

Testimonial: I just wanted to let you know how much I love working out to your tapes. They helped me to alter my physical appearance and increase my self-esteem 100 percent.

Quick Toning Thighs of Steel: The Tamilee Collection

Short on time? No time to work out? Everyone has at least 15 minutes to do some form of exercise. That's what the Quick Toning Tamilee Collection video series is all about. The QT collection gives you a variety of workouts that fit into your hectic schedule. This video consists of three 15-minute workouts focusing on the inner and outer thighs, quadriceps, and hamstrings. This thigh video is one of my favorites. Hope you enjoy it, too.

Quick Toning Upper Body of Steel: The Tamilee Collection

By now you are probably thinking, "When is this woman going to run out of body parts?" This video is also geared for those who don't have much time in their busy schedule to work out, but focuses on the upper body. The three 15-minute workouts consist of one to help you trim your abdominals, one to firm up your chest and back, and one to strengthen and tone your arms. You can get a full upper-body workout with just one videotape.

Quick Toning Lower Body of Steel: The Tamilee Collection

You figured it out (if you read the preceding section): This video covers the other half of your body. Couldn't have guessed it from the name, could you? Similar to the Upper Body of Steel video, this one has three 15-minute workouts focusing on your hips, buns, thighs, and calves. I find that the bottom half of the body is the most popular area for women to work on, but men find these exercises to be extremely beneficial for their buns, too.

Testimonial: I love working out with Tamilee! She is always upbeat, energetic, encouraging, and motivating. I really appreciate the fact that the other people who work out with Tamilee are of different body types and shapes. It makes me feel like I might be considered "normal" after all!

Tamilee's Toning Mind & Body

I'm proud to say this video is one in a series of three where my head isn't cut off for the video box cover. This video in particular is one of my favorites because it is so different from many of the other videos I've done. I truly believe in the mind to muscle connection and using it to help you develop and define your body. The Mind and Body video uses slow, concentrated movements in a variety of standing and floor exercises. You also perform full-body contractions using all the major muscle groups to help you relieve your stress and awaken your senses. Concentrated breathing is emphasized throughout this 30-minute workout. I also show options for exercisers of all fitness levels.

Testimonial: At first I thought it would be difficult, but your words inspired me. . . . Your gift of motivation and inspiration has given me so many things; not only a new shape, but also discipline and a great new attitude towards life.

Tamilee's Building Tighter Assets

This video is your total fitness package. It takes your best asset (your health, not your new car) and makes it better. It's also my first non-Buns of Steel video after a series of 22 videos. This video includes a 30-minute, low-impact step aerobic workout, 30 minutes of muscle shaping exercises for your entire body, and a healthy-eating planner. The bonus planner is filled with delicious recipes and a handy fat calculator to help you determine the best foods to choose when shopping or planning your meals.

Tamilee's Abs Abs Abs

I just can't get enough of those abs, so in this video I decided to spice it up a bit and add two handsome men, each with spectacular six-packs. (You know, those six hard muscles you see when someone has toned abs.) The three of us take you through three 10-minute abdominal workouts. From a classic workout to a super abs workout, you can work your way from beginner to advanced with the on-screen workout level indicator. This fitness indicator shows you when to stop if you are a beginning, intermediate, or advanced exerciser, and continues to motivate you to move to the next level as you progress. In the second and third segments, I include a step to increase the intensity and add variation to the exercises. (Maybe the ab workouts won't be so burdensome for you ladies if you have the help of some men with rippled stomachs coaching you. Or maybe some of you men need competition in order to motivate you.)

Testimonial: Your encouragement provides me with the boost I need to follow my dreams.

Other videos to check out

I would also like to recommend exercise videos from my colleagues who are top fitness instructors in the industry. You can be sure that a video with one of them as an instructor is worth trying out. The instructors listed in the left column offer videos best suited for beginning to intermediate exercisers. If you're looking for a more challenging video that offers intermediate to advanced workouts, try a video from one of these instructors in the right column.

Beginner to intermediate

- Donna Richardson
- Richard Simmons
- Jake Steinfeld's Stretch
- Kathy Smith
- Oprah Winfrey's Make the Connection

Intermediate to advanced

- Karen Voight
- Gin Miller
- The Firm videos
- Kari Anderson
- Crunch videos

Chapter 23
My Ten Favorite Fitness Books

• •

In This Chapter

▶ Healthy books

• •

We live in an age where information is available to us in many ways, shapes, and forms. If you know how to search the Internet, you can find information on just about anything or anybody. But, if you're like me, and you still enjoy old-fashioned book reading, you can still find what you're looking for in a library or a bookstore instead.

Books to Educate and Motivate

Over the years I've compiled a library of wonderful health and fitness books. (I love books; you can usually find me browsing in my local bookstores at least once a week.) The following list shows you some of my favorites. I hope you enjoy them, too!

Anybody's Guide to Total Fitness

Author: Len Kravitz, Ph.D.
Publisher: Kendall/Hunt Publishing Company (1986)
Level: Beginner

Mr. Kravitz is a peer of mine who has been in the health and fitness industry for many years. Although *Anybody's Guide to Total Fitness* is Len's first book, written several years ago, it is an easy-to-read book that includes an illustrated exercise routine. He offers you information on how to start a fitness program, what to wear, and how to set up a home gym, and even includes a trivia quiz. This book is great for first-time exercisers.

Fat to Firm at Any Age

Authors: Alisa Bauman, Sari Harrar, and the editors of Prevention Health Books
Publisher: Rodale Pres, Inc. (1998)
Level: Intermediate

The authors provide you with years of their research — hundreds of interviews conducted with nutritionists, weight loss researchers, exercise physiologists, and fashion designers. This particular book addresses a woman's battle with fat.

Fitness For Dummies

Authors: Suzanne Schlosberg and Liz Neporent, M.A.
Publisher: IDG Books Worldwide, Inc. (1996)
Level: Beginner

This reference book covers it all. Ms. Schlosberg and Ms. Neporent do a superb job of giving their readers a thorough understanding of fitness. If you're confused by all the hype surrounding fitness products, equipment, classes, and weight-loss scams, look through this guide to get answers to all your questions.

How to Lower Your Fat Thermostat

Authors: Dennis Remington, M.D., Garth Fisher Ph.D., and Edward Parent, Ph.D
Publisher: Vitality House International, Inc. (1983)
Level: Advanced

This book was written by three respectable doctors from Brigham Young University and is a great resource for men and women alike. I find the set point theory, which describes how your body gains and loses fat, to be the most interesting portion of this book. These doctors provide an in-depth explanation of the ways in which your hypothalamus controls your body weight and how you can best control it through diet, training, and psychological factors.

If It Hurts, Don't Do It

Authors: Peter Francis, Ph.D. and Lorna Francis, Ph.D.
Publisher: Prima Publishing & Communications (1988)
Level: Beginner to advanced

A husband and wife team, Pete and Lorna are professors at San Diego State University. I have admired them and their work for many years and feel fortunate to have a personal relationship with them and their family. Both Lorna and Pete travel around the world sharing their knowledge of health, fitness, and human mechanics. Their book offers you accurate information and easy-to-follow instructions for self-fitness testing, goal setting, and proper exercise so that you can create the best workout program for your level. It's a must for the beginning exerciser.

Outsmarting the Female Fat Cell

Author: Debra Waterhouse, M.P.H., R.D.
Publisher: Hyperion (1993)
Level: Beginner to advanced

Debra Waterhouse is one of my favorite authors; you can see that I selected two of her books for this chapter. Sometimes I'm asked to speak to groups of people on topics of health and fitness. Most of the time my audience is filled with women who are looking for ways to lose fat and gain muscle. I used this book to formulate my lecture titled, "It's a Matter of Fat." Debra does an excellent job explaining the physiological aspects of a woman's fat cell and how they differ from a man's.

Outsmarting the Mid-Life Fat Cell

Author: Debra Waterhouse, M.P.H., R.D.
Publisher: Hyperion (1998)
Level: Intermediate

If you're a woman approaching mid-life or menopause, and you can't figure out why you're gaining weight, or why you're not losing weight no matter how much you diet and exercise, you need to read this book. Debra takes you through the processes of the female body as it ages, and discusses the societal pressure for women to look good at any age. I recommend this book not only to middle-aged women, but also to young girls. Reading it can help them understand how and why their bodies change as they age and how best to prepare for this natural process of life.

Rubber Band Workout

Author: Tamilee Webb, M.A.
Publisher: Workman Publishing (1986)
Level: Beginner

This is my first book — and it's still going strong today in five countries and four different languages. This book is one of few that is sold with the necessary workout equipment: rubber bands. I demonstrate a variety of exercises for every major muscle group and give options for beginning to advanced exercisers. It makes a great gift for someone who wants to begin exercising at home and has no equipment. If you can stop laughing at my big hairdo and '80s leotard for a moment, you'll get a great workout.

Step Up Fitness Workout

Author: Tamilee Webb, M.A.
Publisher: Workman Publishing (1994)
Level: Beginner

Well, of *course* I'm going to recommend both of my books — I believe in them! *Step Up Fitness Workout* is a great resource for readers who want to learn the basics of step cardio training before they join a class at the gym, or readers who want to have a total body routine to do in the privacy of their own homes. The book is filled with photos and has options for beginning to advanced exercisers, plus bonus exercises for muscle toning using the step.

Science of Stretching

Author: Michael J. Alter
Publisher: Human Kinetics Books (1988)
Level: Advanced

Just as the title states, this book reveals the science behind stretching. It offers readers a very thorough review, but may be a bit technical for beginners. If you're looking for the basics of stretching, start off with Bob Anderson's book *Stretching* (Shelter Publications, 1987).

Fitness via your television

If you can't find what you're looking for in books or videos, try the good old television. Television shows have come a long way. Jack Lalanne introduced us to fitness in the living room and many other fitness celebrities keep us working out there today. Fitness shows can offer a great workout when you don't have time to get to the gym or it's just too cold to exercise outdoors. Today's shows are also geared to educate you. Some shows seem as if their only value is to entertain you with the star's athleticism, but many offer you knowledge of fitness and creative ways to work your body. With all the fitness shows on the air today, you should be able to find a host or a workout that motivates you to move. Grab a tall glass of water and scan your TV channels to check out some of the best fitness motivators in the industry. My first suggestion, of course, is to look for FiT TV, which is the fitness program I co-host with Jake Steinfeld. I was originally offered the chance to help Jake and the Family Channel develop a whole new concept in fitness TV in 1994. FiT TV offers viewers quality health and exercise programming for all levels and all ages and can now be found as a part of the Fox Sports network. You can learn more about FiT TV by checking out the FiT TV Web site (look for the address in Appendix B).

Part VII
Appendixes

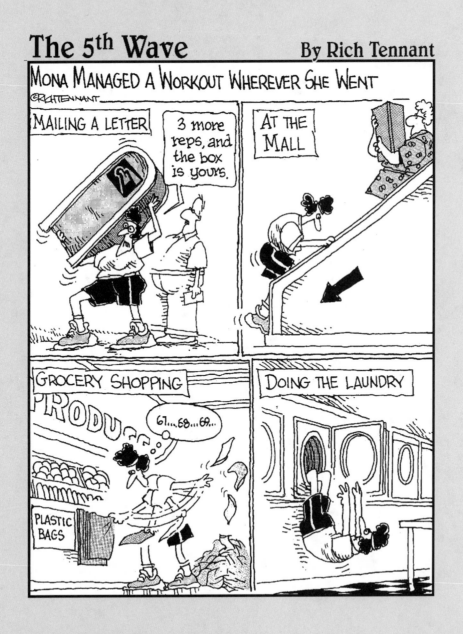

In this part . . .

Here you can find an *Exercise Program Chart* that you can personalize to meet your own needs. I also give you an appendix listing great workout sites on the Web so that you can track down even more resources and information.

Appendix A

Exercise Program Chart

● ●

*Y*ou're on your way to developing your personalized workout program. Before getting started, go through the Home Fitness Evaluation found in Chapter 8. This chapter helps you determine your fitness level as either deconditioned or conditioned. In Chapter 8, I also give you my recommendation on how many sets and repetitions you should perform for each exercise you choose. Repetitions (or reps for short) are the *number of times you perform an exercise* (for example, 10 push-ups). A set is a *group of repetitions,* and I suggest doing 1 to 3 sets of each exercise depending on your level of fitness.

As you look at this chart, you can see that it is separated into parts: one part for your cardiovascular workouts, on which you can find detailed information in Chapter 9, and another part for the muscle-conditioning exercises (found in Chapters 10 through 18). This second part is broken down even further so that each exercise is listed with the chapter number it can be found in (the main chapter for the type of exercise is also given in the heading). All you have to do is highlight your favorites or use the blank spaces to fill in your own favorite exercises and start working out. You may even want to cut your chart out and make copies of it to use as your fitness level progresses.

Cardiovascular (Ch 9)

Activity	Total Time Performed	Distance	Personal Notes
Treadmill			
Jog or run			
Walk			
Bicycle			
Spinning			
Swimming			
Cross-country skiing machine			
Aerobic dance			
Stair climber			
Rowing			
In-line skating			
Other:			

Muscle Toning: Buns (Ch 15)

	Weight	Sets	Reps	Personal Notes
Lunges (Ch 15)				
Rear leg lift (Ch 15)				
Pelvic tilt (Ch 15)				
Chair squat (Ch 17)				
Squat with bar (Ch 17)				
Iso lunge (Ch 17)				
Bun squeezes (Ch 18)				
Sit & stand lift (Ch 18)				
Other:				

Muscle Toning: Legs (Ch 13)

Quadriceps	Weight	Sets	Reps	Personal Notes
Squats (Ch 13)				
Double-leg extension (Ch 13)				
Seated leg extension (Ch 16)				
Seated one-leg extension (Ch 18)				
Seated front-leg lifts with band (Ch 18)				
Other:				

Hamstrings	Weight	Sets	Reps	Personal Notes
One-leg lying heel press (Ch 13)				
One-leg heel curl (Ch 13)				
Hamstring curl (Ch 16)				
Back-thigh curl (Ch 17)				
Standing thigh curl (Ch 18)				
Other:				

Calves	Weight	Sets	Reps	Personal Notes
First-position heel raises (Ch 13)				
Single-heel raises (Ch 13)				
Other:				

Tibia	Weight	Sets	Reps	Personal Notes
Foot taps side to side (Ch 13)				
Ankle circles (Ch 13)				
Other:				

Muscle Toning: Thighs (Ch 14)

Adductors	Weight	Sets	Reps	Personal Notes
Inner-thigh side lift (Ch 14)				
Scissors (Ch 14)				
Pliés (Ch 14)				
Inner-thigh leg lift (Ch 16)				
Seated inner-thigh lift with band (Ch 18)				
Other:				

Abductors	Weight	Sets	Reps	Personal Notes
Lying side leg lifts (Ch 14)				
Standing side leg lifts (Ch 14)				
Side leg lift (Ch 16)				
Outer-thigh press out (Ch 16)				
Leg lifts (Ch 17)				
Seated thigh press out (Ch 18)				
Other:				

Muscle Toning: Back and Shoulders (Ch 11)

Deltoids	Weight	Sets	Reps	Personal Notes
Side raises (Ch 11)				
Rear deltoid lifts (Ch 11)				
Overhead press (Ch 11)				
Shoulder presses (Ch 17)				
Upright rows (Ch 17)				
Other:				

Rotator cuff	Weight	Sets	Reps	Personal Notes
External rotation (Ch 11)				
Internal rotation (Ch 11)				
Other:				

Trapezius	Weight	Sets	Reps	Personal Notes
Shoulder raises (Ch 11)				
Other:				

Rhomboids	Weight	Sets	Reps	Personal Notes
One-arm row (Ch 11)				
Two-arm row (Ch 11)				
Upper-back pullbacks (Ch 16)				
Seated upper-back pullbacks (Ch 18)				
Other:				

Latissimus Dorsi	Weight	Sets	Reps	Personal Notes
Overhead pulldowns (Ch 16)				
Lat stretch (Ch 17)				
Seated one-arm overhead pulldown (Ch 18)				
Other:				

Erector Spinae	Weight	Sets	Reps	Personal Notes
Prone one-leg lift/ Superman (Ch 11)				
Alternate leg lift (Ch 11)				
Other:				

Muscle Toning: Arms and Chest (Ch 10)

Biceps	Weight	Sets	Reps	Personal Notes
Hammer curl (Ch 10)				
Wide curl (Ch 10)				
Alternate curl (Ch 10)				
Front-arm curl (Ch 16)				
Upper-arm curl (Ch 17)				
Seated bicep curl (Ch 18)				
Other:				

Triceps	Weight	Sets	Reps	Personal Notes
Overhead extension (Ch 10)				
Kickbacks (Ch 10)				
Dips (Ch 10)				
Back-arm press down (Ch 16)				
Chair dips (Ch 17)				
Overhead back-arm extension (Ch 17)				
Seated tricep press down (Ch 18)				
Other:				

Chest	Weight	Sets	Reps	Personal Notes
Push-ups (Ch 10)				
Flys (Ch 10)				
Straight-arm pullover (Ch 10)				
Seated chest crossover (Ch 18)				
Other:				

Forearm	Weight	Sets	Reps	Personal Notes
Two-wrist curl-up (Ch 10)				
Two-wrist curl-down (Ch 10)				
Other:				

Muscle Toning: Abdominal (Ch 12)

Abs	Weight	Sets	Reps	Personal Notes
Lower 90-degree contraction (Ch 12)				
Curl-up (Ch 12)				
Crunch (Ch 12)				
Crossover (Ch 12)				
Side lateral slide (Ch 12)				
Ab crunch (Ch 16)				
Chair ab curls (Ch 17)				
Bar crunch (Ch 17)				
Side reaches (Ch 17)				
Seated alternate knee tucks (Ch 18)				
Side ankle touch (Ch 18)				
Seated ab crunch (Ch 18)				
Other:				

Appendix B
Finding Fitness on the Web

· ·

*I*f you're searching for information on fitness, browse the Web for sites that offer products, or look for consumer education organizations. You can find information that ranges from how to become a fitness educator to where to buy the newest fitness products for your home gym.

American College of Sports Medicine

www.acsm.org

This organization publishes a consumer newsletter called *Fitness Matters* that reports on fitness research, equipment, and magazines. The ACSM is one of the most highly regarded organizations in the fitness industry.

Fitness Zone

www.fitnesszone.com

If you're looking for answers to fitness questions, this is your site. You can also share your workout stories and experiences with others in the online chat room.

Fitness Link

www.fitnesslink.com

This service shows you where to go to find solutions to your fitness needs. You can also link up to other fitness organizations through this site.

FiT TV

www.fittv.com

Jake Steinfeld and I host this TV network filled with 20-minute workouts and healthy-living information. You can find more information on how to get this programming by checking out the Web site — and you can get information on the latest fitness information and products on the market, as well.

SPRI Products

www.fitnessonline.com/shop/SPRI

If you are interested in purchasing the rubber exercise products I use in this book, check out SPRI Web site. You can also send for a catalog of all their products and videos from this site, or call 800-222-7774.

Lasting Results

www.lastingresults.com

This Web site is full of great information. You can find a full-body muscle-conditioning workout that has a demonstration of each exercise with moving figures. You can see how the exercise is performed with perfect form. You'll also find a section that lists common questions with the answers. Leave your own question and e-mail address for a personal answer.

Tamilee Webb

www.tamileewebb.com

Stop by and visit my site. If you are interested in a video, have questions to ask, or are just looking for some fitness information, look up my site and say hello.

Index